LOVE, SEX AND POWER
IN LATER LIFE

FREEDOM PRESS publishes *Freedom* fortnightly, *The Raven* quarterly, and anarchist books and pamphlets (currently sixty five titles in print).

Freedom is a propaganda newspaper, commenting on world affairs from an anarchist point of view. The first edition appeared in October 1886. Its style has always been discursive, seeking to disseminate anarchism by getting anarchist ideas discussed by readers outside the anarchist movement.

The Raven is a quarterly magazine of 96 pages, dealing with anarchist ideas at greater length. Recent issues have included collections of essays on Education, Revolution, Communication and Health.

Freedom Press has published books and pamplets for more than a century. These include classic and recent statements of the anarchist case, history books, hilarious cartoon books, and anarchist treatments of particular aspects of life. The Anarchist Discussion series was begun in 1991.

Freedom Press is European distributor for some North American anarchist publishers and distributes many anarchist publications in the English Language.

Freedom Press Bookshop, open six days a week, also sells works of anarchist interest from commercial and academic publichers, across the counter and by mail order. The shop entrance is in Angel Alley, a long passage approached by a pedestrian tunnel, alongside the Whitechapel Art Gallery.

Send for a free specimen copy of *Freedom* and a list of over 400 titles, most of them post free:

Freedom Press, 84b Whitechapel High Street, London, E1 7QX.

LOVE, SEX AND POWER IN LATER LIFE

A *Libertarian Perspective*

by

TONY GIBSON

FREEDOM PRESS
1992

Published by
FREEDOM PRESS
84b Whitechapel High Street
London, E1 7QX

© Tony Gibson and Freedom Press 1992

ISBN 0 900384 65 4

Printed by
Aldgate Press, 84b Whitechapel High Street, London, E1 7QX

CONTENTS

Introduction

Those of us who have lived as mature adults over the past 30 years have witnessed a virtual revolution in sexual mores in Western Europe and most of the developed world, despite lack of social progress in many other important areas. A number of related factors brought the question of love and sex into prominence in the post-war era. The stimulating, if sometimes excessively wild and speculative writings of Wilhelm Reich and his followers brought to the notice of the Left, how sexual behaviour was related to libertarian politics, and FREEDOM PRESS distributed his books. FREEDOM PRESS still stocks *Sexpol: Essays 1929-34*[1], which reprints some of the best essays of Wilhelm Reich.

It is difficult for younger people in the 1990s to appreciate the severity of the general sexual repression that existed in Britain in the immediate post-war era of the 1940s. The great lexicographer Eric Partridge in his scholarly tome *A Dictionary of Slang and Unconventional English* naturally had to deal with the word "fuck", its etymology and usage, but he could not print the word. We therefore have a long and scholarly discourse on f***, f***ing, f***ed, f***er etc., which now seems to us quite ridiculous. In Partridge's *A Dictionary of the Underworld* the word does not appear at all, although he risks a mention of "c –" among his "low slang". In this prudish climate, people who lived in bed-sitters generally couldn't risk having a member of the opposite sex visiting them in their room, even at tea-time, although there was some latitude which was class-linked; that is, a middle-class landlady might allow her middle-class male lodger to have a girl-friend to tea, but a working-class landlady would not. As one such woman said to me, "I'm either keeping one sort of house or another – and I'm not keeping that sort of house!" However, the repressive sexual mores of the hypocritical Victorian era which had lingered on were breaking down, and the social upheaval of two world wars had contributed to the liberalization of attitudes, and permitted pioneering researchers such as Kinsey and his associates to attempt to study human sexuality objectively – against a howl of protest from some quarters. I will discuss the Kinsey studies later on.

Wilhelm Reich

Reich is important because he was one of the first to see clearly how sexual repression is linked to political and social repression. He graduated in Medicine in Vienna in the 1920s and became a protege of Sigmund Freud, becoming influential in the psycho-analytic movement of the time. Unlike most of the psychoanalysts, he was politically conscious and was active in the Austrian Socialist Party, but eventually he joined the Communist Party and moved to Berlin. There, he was a member of a cell that contained other comrades who, after they had broken with the Party, became quite famous, including Arthur Koestler, the novelist and para-psychology freak. Reich's best-known book, *The Mass Psychology of Fascism*[2], set out his basic thesis: the sexual frustration of the proletariat prevented them from ever growing up properly; thus they failed to attain political maturity and consciousness of their true personal dignity, value and power. Although Reich put forward his thesis in Marxist terms, referring to the fiction of "the proletariat", there is obviously a great deal of truth in his contention. The individual who doesn't fulfil his or her sexual potential lacks an essential component of what makes for autonomy and a sense of personal worth. This has been recognized since the earliest times; thus male calves are castrated so that they will develop into patient working oxen and not fiery and unmanageable bulls, and some despotic cultures have castrated their young slaves so that they will become patient drudges who never rise in rebellion. To this thesis, Reich added a curious rider that what was utterly essential in the expression of sexuality was the attainment of orgasm, although he never clarified what he meant by orgasm, and later work in sexology has shown how muddled he was in this concept.

In *The Mass Psychology of Fascism* Reich argued that the German Nazis, and all fascists in general, were the victims of extreme sexual repression and immaturity, and that however much they strove to present a dominant and macho image, they were really cringing inadequates who worshipped the boot that kicked them hardest. He wrote:

German fascism made an all-out effort to anchor itself in the psychic structures of the masses and therefore placed the greatest emphasis upon the inculcation of the adolescents and children. It had no other means at its disposal than the rousing and cultivation of slavery to authority, the basic precondition of which is ascetic, sex-negating education. The natural sexual strivings towards the other sex, which seek gratification from childhood on, were replaced in the main by distorted and diverted homosexual and sadistic feelings, and in part also by asceticism. This applies, for instance, in the so-called esprit de corps that was cultivated in the Labour Conscription Camps, as well as the so-called 'spirit of discipline and obedience' which was preached everywhere. The hidden motive behind these slogans was to unleash brutality and make it ready for use in imperialistic wars. Sadism originates from ungratified orgastic yearnings[3].

Again, there is a lot of truth in this, and the idea was taken up in the U.S.A. by Adorno and his colleagues, who were mostly Jewish refugees from Nazi oppression, and their researches were published as *The Authoritarian Personality*[4], not a very impressive work that leans too heavily on much psychoanalytic speculation.

Not only did Reich have to leave Germany in 1933 as a Jew and an outspoken critic of the Nazis who had newly come to power, but his writings were condemned by the Red Pope in Moscow as being "un-Marxist rubbish". So he left the Communist Party. He was also expelled from the International Psychoanalytic Association, who had their own Pope in Vienna, who would tolerate no deviation from the orthodox doctrine which was as fundamentally bourgeois as its founder. Thus Reich was on his own, the victim of real persecution and, in his later years, paranoid delusions of grandeur, mixed with ideas of continued persecution from unlikely quarters. Like most psychoanalysts, he had no grasp of scientific method, and even in his earlier works that have some value, there are many signs of his mistaking personal speculation for established fact. Most of his later writings, when he was living in Cloud Cuckoo Land in the U.S.A, that embarrassed his more intelligent followers, are hardly worth mentioning, but it is of interest to note that his earlier writings which Marie Louise Berneri obtained with some difficulty in the 1940s to distribute through Freedom Press, and which seemed so revolutionary in the 1940s, are now published in paperback by Penguin Books and are quite unremarkable in the climate of opinion today. At least Reich had the germ of an important idea, dismissed as "un-Marxist rubbish" by Moscow, but taken up by the anarchist movement which developed it further.

The Anarchist Contribution to Sexual Emancipation

The movement for emancipation from Victorian repression was not wholly dominated by Reich and his followers. There had been plenty of currents of opinion in Britain that far ante-dated Reich's writings. World War I had been instrumental in advancing the status of women, for girls got away from the stultifying domination of the paternalistic family to work in the Land Army, nursing abroad, and other war-work which demanded their services, and the later war continued this process.

Victorian prudery was supported by the grossest of male hypocrisy. It used to be held that "nice" women didn't enjoy sexual intercourse and participated in it only for the purpose of pleasing their husbands and for the sake of bearing children. This attitude was seriously supported by much orthodox medical opinion, and one marriage manual stated the following:

> As a general rule, a modest woman seldom desires any sexual gratification for herself. She submits to her husband, but only to please him; and, but for the desire for maternity, would far rather be relieved from his attentions.[5]

Perry London describes the Victorian ideal of what a wife should be, and writes:

> The Victorian wife was to be sweet-tempered, docile, adoring and utterly subservient to her husband, who was to dominate the relationship in all respects. Neither admitted to any sexual feelings, and the more "pure" their love, the less lustful it was presumed to be. Wifely modesty required the wearing of copious garments, never exposing the body naked (not to physician, not to husband), never naming body parts or functions, never showing passion in the sex act. By and large the husband reciprocated in modesty and language, and did his "connubial duty" quickly and silently[6].

Despite this totally unreal picture of womanhood that was maintained by the male establishment and unthinkingly accepted by girls brought up in appalling ignorance, London was the brothel capital of Europe, and every variety of prostitution was available for those who could pay. We hear a lot nowadays about the age-old practice of child sex abuse, a matter that appears to titillate the fantasy of some types of do-gooders and evangelical religious cranks[7], but it is nothing compared with the extent of enforced juvenile prostitution that flourished in the latter part of Queen Victoria's reign, and was winked at by outwardly respectable people.

Women in the anarchist movement have always taken a strongly feminist position, although traditionally it has been different from the stance taken by the lesbian-feminists of today. Pioneers such as Rose Witcop and Lilian Wolfe asserted their individuality by refusing to marry their lovers at a time when "living in sin" was regarded as disgraceful for women, and younger generations of women have benefited from their example without, perhaps, fully realizing the enormous pressures, both social and economic, that these women fought against.

In the 1940s, anarchist writers such as John Hewetson[8], Alex Comfort[9], Philip Sansom[10] and myself[11] lectured and wrote articles and pamphlets about sexual emancipation for the anarchist press and in liberal journals such as Norman Haire's *Journal of Sex Education*[12]. Much of this seems rather dated when read today, for such educative efforts were partially responsible for what has been termed "the sexual revolution", a radical change of social attitudes towards sexuality that occured in the 1950s and 1960s, and affected both law and common practice.

Looking back at our early publications, it is apparent that what we were chiefly concerned with was the emancipation of *the young* from the irrational and repressive control of the law, and the older generations who were still steeped in the Victorian taboos that had so often warped their own lives. We were quite young ourselves, and reacting against what we had had to struggle against in our earlier years. Now, 40 years later, a very different situation exists, which is well expressed by a writer to *The Lancet*:

> the younger generation, so liberal, so free, so uninhibited by old-fashioned conventions according to themselves, are often rigid, narrow, puritanical, and censorious when it comes to the behaviour of the older citizens[13].

This, of course, relates to the question of a conflict of power between the older and younger generations, a question that will be explored later in this book. The kernel of truth that lies in Reich's contention that the ruling class would like to "castrate", in a figurative sense, the proletariat, can be applied to the situation in which some of the younger generations would like to regard "the old" as being asexual and impotent in every sense, and fit only to drag out the miserable remainder of their years on a wretched pension, divorced from the real concerns of life, until they thankfully drop dead. There is a huge folk-lore about "the old" that can be invoked to make them feel ashamed of being other than harmless old dodderers. Older men who continue to show a normal adult sexual interest are characterized as "dirty old men", and older women who continue to seek an active sex-life are similarly stigmatized and called by nasty names. In many respects, the old are the gaolers of the old: it's they who pass on the inherited repressive tradition. This mirrors the classic view of class-struggle in which the active lower ranks of the oppressors of the poor are drawn from the proletariat themselves: the police, gendarmerie, prison screws and military being working-class men and women.

We mustn't over-generalize and imply that all younger and middle-aged people are engaged in a deliberate attempt to denigrate and put down those over the age of retirement. Personally I have the highest regard for the younger generations who have successfully thrown off the tyranny of the Marxist-Leninist regimes that my own generation tolerated for too long. However, "ageism", like "racism" and "sexism" is often unthinkingly applied in making judgements and implementing policies, because it is imbedded in the traditional zeitgeist.

The Kinsey Studies and After.

In the post-war era the studies of Kinsey[14] produced quite a revolution in thinking about the sex-lives of young and middle-aged adults, and the re-adjustment of social values led to the later inquiries of a more detailed nature, notably the clinical studies of Masters and Johnson[15]. But in these researches it was taken for granted that it was hardly worth while questioning men and women over the age of 60, for as such older people seldom used to consult their doctors about sexual problems, it was assumed that normal older people were totally uninterested in sex.

In the 1970s plenty of different sorts of books dealing with sex were published, and much of the older folk-lore that served earlier repressive attitudes was denied. Alex Comfort, no longer an obscure anarchist writer, hit the jackpot with his *Joy of Sex* and *More Joy of Sex*. But most of these books hardly touched on the love and sex-lives of oldsters. Towards the end of that decade, however, a lot more information about the sex-lives of older people began to be published. There was the Starr-Weiner Report[16] published in 1981, and Edward Brecher's study for the American Consumers' Association, reporting on the sex-lives of 4,246 men and women aged between 50 and 93, was published in 1984[17]. These books certainly were an eye-opener! We now recognize that many normal men and women in their 60s, 70s. 80s, and older do indeed have significant sex lives both emotionally and physically, although expressed rather differently than in their younger years. The facts that have emerged surprised many people. When people reach an age that society designates as "old" many are themselves surprised to find that they don't feel any different, except for an inevitable waning of their physical robustness.

Older men and women who find that they still have the same emotional and physical reactions sexually, may privately regard themselves as being rather "odd", and may not realize that they are entirely normal; but when they're lucky enough to meet others in their age-group who feel just the same, then they begin to discover that ageing as such needn't make a very great difference. If such realization is achieved, it produces a great increase in self-confidence, and heartens people to live fuller lives in every respect in their later years, and to stand up for their rights, as manifest in such organizations as The Grey Panthers. We don't yet know much about the relationship of continued health and longevity to emotional and sexual satisfaction in the later years, but there are some encouraging pointers.

The Issues Discussed in the Present Book.

The anarchist movement has always put forward the case for getting the best out of our lives, and struggling against social forces of every kind that would deny us. This struggle doesn't cease at any age in life, and it is false to imagine that it's inevitable that we become more conservative and less revolutionary with age. Love and sex play an important part in the lives of most men and women, and there is no reason at all why this shouldn't be so however long we live. Of course our physical prowess declines with age, but the emotional side of our being need not change. Indeed, Bashevis Singer, the well-known Yiddish writer, holds that, "In love, as in other matters, the young are just beginners". With the power to love goes the power to struggle in a personal and social sense, and as we age we should use our collective experience to recognize mistakes of the past, and to bring about social change.

In the present book a good deal of relevant factual information is presented. Where appropriate, readers are referred to proper scientific sources. The processes of ageing are described with regard to emotional and sexual fulfilment, and problems both psychological and physical are examined, with advice for over-coming them. The present-day social attitudes towards love and sex in later life are examined, and the case is made for modifying them, and making all doctors and other professionals who have a responsibility towards older people more aware of the facts that have come to light as the result of recent research, challenging the traditional repressive assumptions that are held by all too many conservative medical practitioners and social workers. The image that many older people have of themselves is fully discussed and questioned, and it is proposed that many problems encountered will disappear when people adopt a new concept of sexuality appropriate to their age. The book goes on to discuss the whole question of the attitude of younger people, some of whom are dominated by property-conscious expectations of inheritance, and actually jealous sexually of the continued love-lives of people in their families who are much older. The special emotional problems that ageing brings to both sexes are examined, with particular emphasis being laid on the dilemma of older women who are apt to suffer from the double hazards of ageism and sexism.

The final chapter of the book projects into the future and discusses probable changes in society which will naturally follow from the radical alteration in the population structure that has occurred, and which will be exaggerated as time goes on. These include changes in the balance of power between the young and the old, and the relations between men and women in their later years. The ideas of Wilhelm Reich are again discussed, and it is suggested that the large and significant section of the population who are now over the official age of retirement can be considered as a new "class", and the classic ideas of class-struggle and challenging the dominant ideology are examined in relation to this new concept. By facing these issues now we may affect the future for younger generations.

Introduction: Notes

1. Wilhelm Reich, *Sexpol: Essays 1929-34*. Random House, 1972.

3. Wilhelm Reich, *The Mass Psychology of Fascism*. Penguin Books, 1970

3. Ibid.

4. T.W. Adorno et al., *The Authoritarian Personality*. Harper, 1950.

5. Cited by R.N. Butler & M.I. Lewis, *Love and Sex After 60* Harper & Row, 1988.

6. Perry London, "Sexual behavior". In W.T. Reich (ed.), *Encyclopedia of Bioethics*. The Free Press, 1978.

7. Donald Rooum, "The satanic child abuse epidemic, 1990-91". *The R a v e n*, 1991, 15, 245-250.

8. John Hewetson, *Sexual Freedom for the Young: Society and the Sexual Life of Children and Adolescents*. Freedom Press, 1951.

9. Alex Comfort, *Barbarism and Sexual Freedom*. Freedom Press, 1948.

10. Philip Sansom, "Discussion of the Blackpool obscenity trial". *Journal of Sex Education*, 3, 160-161,1951.

11. Tony Gibson, *Youth for Freedom*. Freedom Press, 1948.

12. The four anarchist writers referred to above contributed various articles, both singly and in controversy, in the *Journal of Sex Education* during the five years of its existence 1948-1952.

13. In England Now, *The Lancet* 1986, January 18th, 147.

14. A.C. Kinsey et al., *Sexual Behavior in the Human Male*. 1948: *Sexual Behavior in the Human Female*. 1953. W.B. Saunders.

15. W.H. Masters & V.E. Johnson, *Human Sexual Response*. Little, Brown & Co., 1966. *Human Sexual Inadequacy*. J.A. Churchill, 1970.

16. B.D. Starr & M.B. Weiner, *The Starr-Weiner Report on Sex and Sexuality in the Mature Years*. McGraw Hill, 1981.

17. E.M. Brecher, Love, Sex and Aging: A Consumer Union Report. Little, Brown & Co., 1984

Physical Changes in Sexual Capacity and Experience with Ageing: The Myths and the Reality

As mentioned in the introduction, the idea that "old" people are, or should be, without sexual drive and capacity serves the function of jockeying them into a relatively powerless position in society. They are regarded as "past it", and consequently not of fully adult status,to be pitied and patronized. This myth is an ancient one, and finds expression in our literature. Thus Shakespeare's Hamlet lectured his mother Gertrude (who can only have been in her 40s!) thus:

> O shame! Where is thy blush? Rebellious hell,
> If thou canst mutine in a matron's bones
> To flaming youth let virtue be as wax,
> And melt in her own fire: proclaim no shame
> When the compulsive ardour gives the charge,
> Since frost itself as actively doth burn,
> And reason panders will.

But all his mother was doing was going to bed with her new husband Claudius; Hamlet was consumed with sexual jealousy, all the worse because he was not having a fulfilled relationship with Ophelia for various neurotic reasons, and suspecting that Claudius had killed his father. One can find plenty of other examples in literature of "old" people being reproved or mocked because they showed sexual interest: the Merry Wives of Windsor (a right pair of cock-teasers) led Falstaff on in order to humiliate him; Chaucer's "old" knight January (he was only 60) being mocked and cuckolded for marrying young May; Congreve's Lady Wishfort being ridiculed for her sexual interest in Mirabel, in *The Way of the World.*

Undoubtedly the strength of the sexual impulse does get less with age, and in fact it begins to decline in men after the age of about 20 according to Kinsey. But how do we measure "strength"? In number of orgasms per week, which appears to have been Kinsey's measure for males? This is a somewhat unsatisfactory yardstick, as more mature males often cultivate delaying and controlling the seminal emission as part of a sophisticated technique of lovemaking. And for women, if we simply count the number of times they copulate per week, this leaves out of account the sexual capacity of their partners, and, more importantly, how satisfying these sexual acts are for them. Perhaps we are on the wrong track if we seek to quantify sexual drive in terms of these crude physiological measures. First, it may be useful if we list the widespread myths about sexuality and ageing, as set out in Table 1.

Table 1.

Myths about sexuality and ageing.

1. Intercourse and emission of semen are debilitating and will tend to hasten old age and death.

2. One's sex life can be prolonged by abstinence in earlier years and inactivity in later years.

3. Masturbation is a childish activity that is put aside when one reaches, adulthood, and is carried out by older persons only if they are seriously disturbed.

4. Coital satisfaction decreases considerably after the menopause.

5. Older men are particularly subject to sexual deviations, for example, exhibitionism and child molesting.

6. Older women who still enjoy sex were probably nymphomaniacs when they were younger.

7. Most older men lose their ability and desire to have sex.

8. Sexual ability and performance remain the same throughout life.

9. If older individuals go without sex for several years, they will not be able to have sex at a future time.

10. Older people with chronic illness or physical disabilities should cease sex activity completely.

Croft, L.H. (1982) *Sexuality in Later Life.* Appendix B. Boston: JohnWright.

Because of the prevalence of these myths, it will be helpful to deal with them in some detail, and make a brief reference to some of the scientific evidence in the Notes.

1. All that we know about the physiology of sex makes it quite clear that intercourse and the emission of semen is not debilitating. In later life, men do not manufacture as much semen, just as some other natural secretions are not as copious, and some acts of intercourse are not accompanied by a seminal emission. Nonetheless, they may still have an orgasm, which is an event in the nervous system, and experience the pleasure and relaxation that follows. What evidence we have shows that continued sexual activity is associated with longevity, and it may be that the former promotes the latter[1].

2. This is simply rubbish.

3. Some people masturbate all their lives, whether or not they are also engaging in sex with a partner. Masturbation is almost universalamong males, particular when they are young, lusty and lacking sexual partners. Some females claim that they never, or very rarely, masturbate. Many older people who have not got partners masturbate regularly, and it is a healthful way of relieving sexual tension[2].

4. For some women the menopause causes a severe deficiency of the hormone oestrogen, and this can cause vaginal dryness and hence pain on intercourse. This can be remedied by hormone replacement therapy, a sophisticated treatment that needs medical monitoring, and in a few cases is not advisable[3]. But for a number of other women pleasure in intercourse increases after the menopause, largely for psychological reasons, such as ceasing to have to bother about contraception, and leading a more relaxed style of life because their children are grown up[4].

5. This is quite untrue, yet the myth was perpetuated even by such a relatively enlightened sexologist as Havelock Ellis. Child molesters are typically males in their thirties whose sex-lives have been warped and stunted by a moralistic upbringing[5]

6. The term "nymphomaniac" is a silly term of abuse applied to women who enjoy sex and rival men in their ability to go out and get it. Most older women enjoy sex, the tragedy is that for social and demographic reasons many of them are without partners in the later years of life[6].

7. This is not true. Various surveys involving thousands of older men show that the great majority of older men are interested in sex. Their "ability" in terms of penile potency, declines with age, just as their ability to run round the block and other physical achievements decline[7]

8. Of course they don't, and anyone in their seventies who thinks that they "ought" to function, in a physical sense, as they did in their twenties, is a fool. We function *differently* when we are older, and some people say that their sex-lives are better in later life[8].

9. In general, this is not true, but if individuals have become discouraged and believe themselves to be "past it", they may have difficulty in resuming a sex-life for psychological reasons even when an opportunity occurs. A lot depends upon one's self-image.

10. The fear of doing oneself an injury by copulating is common. On the contrary, the maintenance of sexual activity keeps up the morale of a sick or injured person and responsible authorities have been concerned with advising handicapped and sick people how best they may adapt to their disabilities and continue to make love[9].

A General Overview.

Having disposed of the common myths about sex and ageing, let us now consider what really does happen to the sexuality of men and women as they age. First, it should be noted that there are enormous differences between individuals in this matter. Kinsey noted that it was impossible to say what sexual practices, frequencies, etc. were "normal" as people varied so greatly. This is especially true with regard to age, some fifty-year-olds apparently running out of steam while other people in their nineties are still making love.

It will be convenient to consider the effect of the ageing process for the two sexes separately. Men tend to suffer from an over-emphasis on physical prowess all their lives; as they age they become less athletic, and this, of course, is manifest in their sexual behaviour as well as everything else.. According to Butler & Lewis, "Most men begin to worry secretly about sexual ageing some time in their thirties, when they compare their present level of sexual activity with their previous performance as teenagers and very young adults."[10] I must say that this surprises me, but as these authors are writing about the American scene I'll take their word for it. One change that takes place is that the male orgasm does not take place so quickly, but for most couples I would think that this is a positive advantage, since the act of copulation may be prolonged by the older man, giving his partner repeated orgasms if this is desired. Because, as pointed out above, people vary so enormously in their love-making style, no-one can compare himself with a given norm; all he can do is to compare his present with his past performance. If he is made aware of a general truth – that lovemaking in one form or another generally continues for the whole of a man's life, if he feels like it, then he will be re-assured and will not become prey to neurotic anxiety. In his teens he may have liked to have it off three times a night, and now in his forties he only has it three times a week – but does it matter? Is he really getting less satisfaction out of his sex-life? It may be that the three times a night performance was really to show his girl-friend what a hell of fine stud he was, but now 25 years later, he's more secure in his masculine role and doesn't need to show off, and really gives himself and his partner more satisfaction than in his teen-age years. When he's in his seventies, a week or more may sometimes pass without a single act of intercourse, but he may still make love in other ways, such love-making being a steady part of an on-going erotic love-relationship. His masculine self-image suffers no diminution because he makes love like a seventy-year-old and not like a teenager, when it was all "Wham-bam -goodbye ma'm!".

A ribald joke relates how a sex researcher was lecturing, and having ascertained that every single member of the audience was currently having a sex-life, began to ask about frequencies. "Seven nights a week?" Three hands went up. "Four or more times a week?" Twelve hands went up. "Once or twice a week?" Twenty hands went up. And so it went on, just one individual indicating that he had it only once a month. But the lecturer noticed that in the front there was a grinning individual who had never put up his hand at all. "You sir, you seem very pleased with yourself, but I didn't see you raise your hand at all. Tell me, please, how frequently do you have intercourse?" "Once a year," the happy man replied, "But it's tonight!"

If men are ignorant about what will happen to them as they get older they may make both themselves and their partners miserable about sex, give the whole thing up, and be reconciled to being pathetic old sex-less dodderers retired from the battle of life. Let us consider the views of Fred, a hypothetical character just turned seventy:

"What – Charley down the road running after that red-headed widow is he? He's nothing but a dirty old man. I ain't had a bit of grumble for twenty years or more – don't expect to at my age. My old woman 'ud have a fit if I suggested it.   No – beer's my pleasure".

But if any men in their seventies expect to continue to lead the same sort of sex-life that they did in their forties they will be sadly disappointed, and if they don't realize the normal age-related changes that take place in both men and women, they will become very inadequate lovers. In general, elderly people don't expect to continue to make love in the same way as they did in middle-age, but they're often very unsure as to what will happen. Some men fear that they will become impotent after the age of about 50 or 60, and here they may be a prey to some scare advertising that has been appearing in the press very recently. A commercial firm that advertises its services for preserving or restoring potency makes the following misleading statement in its publicity brochure:

> Thanks to a revolutionary breakthrough male impotence can now be successfully treated in nine cases out of ten. This distressing condition is more common than most people imagine. Ten per cent of all men are affected and up to 40% of those over the age of 50.

This is scare advertising, intended to frighten people into coming for treatment and paying out big fees. To claim that "ten per cent of all men are affected" is virtually meaningless. First, they don't define "impotence"; failure to achieve or maintain erection on all occasions, or one occasion in ten, or one in 100? Second, to say that "up to 40% of those over the age of 50", are affected, is rubbish. What does "up to" mean? The percentage affected depends upon the particular age cohort that is being studied. Finally, it is absurd to make a claim that successful treatment can be given to "nine cases out of ten". This certainly wouldn't be true if all their clients were in their 90s! The treatment this clinic offers, according to their publicity brochure, is "Pharmacologically Induced Penile Erection" which probably means the injection of papavervine or similar agents into the penis, a technique that may have considerable dangers, and may need continued expensive medical monitoring.[11]

Men who don't properly understand what's happening to them in the normal course of ageing, may fear that they are becoming impotent simply because they experience one or two incidents of failure toachieve erection on a sexual encounter. Such a fear may very well produce performance anxiety which can cause psychogenic impotence. But occasional incidents of unexplained failure to achieve erection happen to some people at all ages, and do not mean very much. Ovid, the great Latin poet of love and sexual technique wrote an amusing poem on the subject. No doubt advertisers of commercial treatments such as that mentioned above, hope to attract such cases as clients.

Not only do men need know what physiological changes they may expect to take place in their own bodies, and how to cope with them, but they need to understand what happens to women in order to be effective and considerate lovers. Most men probably underestimate the capacity for enjoyment and sexual performance in older women. They are aware that their own sexual performance is declining, and so expect a comparable decline to take place in women, which is not the case. They may not know that if a decline in sexual capacity in women follows the menopause, this may be due to a lack of the hormone oestrogen, a condition that can generally be rectified quite easily by hormone replacement therapy. As mentioned before, some women enjoy sex more after the menopause.

Women also need to know about men. In their younger years they may have come to regard men as robust and ever-ready studs, who could be expected to do all the wooing to bring on the conventionally reluctant female. In later life the roles may become somewhat reversed in this respect, the sexuality of the woman being the more robust, and that of the man more subject to subtle psychological influences. Sometimes the sex instruction manuals that are written for younger adults make statements that aren't quite true for older people. Thus Williams states that "A woman's desire and responsiveness tends to be even more susceptible to psychological influences, internal and external, than a man's. As the saying goes, 'Biology moves her but psychology rules her!'"[12]. Allowing for the fact that there are enormous individual differences, this male/female contrast is less true in later life, and in many cases the reverse is true, older women being tougher. They live, on average, seven years longer than men, are less upset by bereavement of a spouse, and their sexual capacity doesn't decline with age to the same extent as men's. Their trouble is that there just aren't enough men in their age-group, and many of those who are around are just too timorous and emotionally feeble to play a proper masculine part.

Above we envisaged the hypothetical Fred, who gave up love-making because he felt that he couldn't live up to his previous standards of performance. This creates a most unfortunate social situation. If older men fear the "challenge" of a situation in which their sexual potency will be put to the test, then they may withdraw from socialization with women, as well as from sexual encounters with them, and this exacerbates a problem that already exists – that there are already four times as many *single* women as *single* men after the age of 65. Unless both men and women in the later years of life have adequate knowledge about sexuality, the relations between the two sexes are beset with pitfalls – pitfalls that have been created by the Victorian anti-sex tradition, and the power struggle that seeks to relegate "the old" to an inferior position in society. This is not a sex-instruction manual; readers who want to gain more knowledge of the subject are referred to Appendix 1. .

Chapter 1: Notes

1. The question of longevity and sexuality is dealt with in detail in Chapter 4.

2. Starr & Weiner (op. cit. Introduction) asked their 443 respondents the question, "Do you masturbate?"; for men, 52.6% of the 60-69 age group, and 32.7% of the 70+ group replied "Yes", a drop of nearly 20% with ageing. For women, there was no such significant drop with ageing, the relevant percentages being 41.1% and 46.8%. In Brecher's study (op. cit.) the drop in frequency of masturbation was far more pronounced in men than in women. Starr and Weiner's data are also of interest in that they show that although the difference in the incidence of female masturbation is in the expected direction, there is not a great deal of difference between the married, widowed, divorced and single women, indicating that it is not simply a practice engendered by sexual privation.

3. For up to date details about hormone replacement therapy, see W.H. Utian "Analysis of hormone replacement therapy". In J.W.W. Studd & M.I. Whitehead, (eds.) *The Menopause*. Blackwell Scientific Publications, 1988.

4. The 441 women over 60 in the Starr-Weiner survey were asked"How does sex feel now compared with when you were younger?". In their responses 41.0% reported "better", 39.7% reported "the same",and 19.3% said it was "worse". Lesser satisfaction was expressed by men.

5. I have discussed the extraordinary misinformation perpetuated by Havelock Ellis in my book *The Emotional and Sexual Lives of OlderPeople*, Chapter 1. (H.B. Gibson, Chapman & Hall, 1991). See the following information about child molesters: Pedophiles tend to be rigidly religious and moralistic. As with most aberrant sexual behaviors that have been described, there is a strong subjective feeling in the compulsion that draws the pedophile to the

child..... The pedophiles ... were found to cluster into three age groups,adolescence, mid-to-late thirties, and mid to late fifties, with the mid-thirties group the largest. (G.C. Davison & J.M. Neale, *AbnormalPsychology*. p.227. Wiley & Sons, 1974).

6. The question of the numerical imbalance between the sexes, and its consequences, is discussed in Chapter 8.

7. See Edwin Brecher's study of 2,402 males. In their 50s, 98% said they were sexually active; in their 60s, 91% claimed activity; for those70+, 79% claimed activity. Not much lack of interest here!

8. This matter will be clarified when we discuss the more sophisticated forms of lovemaking that are enjoyed in later life, in Chapter 5.

9. See R.N. Butler & M.I. Lewis, (op. cit. Introduction). See also, L. Katzin, "Chronic illness and sexuality". *American Journal of Nursing*, 1990, January, 56-59.

10. R.N.Butler & M.I.Lewis, op. cit.

11. See W.R. Guirguis, "The use and abuse of intercavernous injectionof vasoactive drugs" *British Journal of Sexual Medicine* 1989, 16,9-11

12. W. Williams *Man, Woman and Sexual Desire*. Williams & Wilkins, 1986.

Repressive Social Attitudes Towards Sexuality in Later Life

I t is maintained in this book that there is a strongly negative attitude towards the sexual activity of people who are designated as "elderly", and it is suggested that this parallels the Reichian thesis that the ruling class seeks to deny sexual freedom to the governed as a means of keeping them in immaturity and powerlessness. We do not have to prove that this is a matter of a consciously worked out strategy; it is merely a traditional policy, just like the fostering of religion, whether it is Christian, Islamic, or Marxist, to keep the masses in subjection.

It may be objected that anti-sexual attitudes are merely part of our tradition, and that although the young have thrown off the yoke of repression to a great degree, the old simply haven't had the energy or inclination to follow suit, largely because they are "past it" anyway. However, it should be pointed out that those who are now in the age cohorts of the sixties and seventies, were young adults who accomplished the "sexual revolution" in the post-Kinsey era. In the previous chapter it was shown that elderly people are certainly not "past it" in a physical sense, but that the barriers to the continued enjoyment of a satisfying sex-life in later life are largely psychological. What needs to be demonstrated is that there is a very definite tendency to denigrate older people simply on the grounds of their age, and to force on them a stereotype that denies them their full rights as citizens.

Much of the social science that has been directed towards ousting older people from adequate power in society, goes by the name of "disengagement theory"[1]. Much what was written about the disengagement of older people in the sociological and developmental literature some time ago was based on a self-fulfilling prophecy: they have been compelled to disengage because of the social and economic pressures that have been put upon them, yet this isn't an entirely modern phenomenon. The fate of Shakespeare's King Lear, who felt that he should disengage in favour of his daughters, should be a warning to us all!

Disengagement theory holds that the process of giving up rights and responsibilities at a certain age, and retiring to a metaphorical rocking chair, is universal, and moreover, that it's to the advantage of both society and the individual. It hardly needs pointing out that a neurosurgeon can't operate as effectively in his 50s as when he was younger, just as a coal-heaver can' t heave coal as efficiently after a certain age, but that doesn't mean that they must necessarily disengage either socially, economically or sexually as they age and be reconciled to living on a pittance, accepting a less respected place in society, and be content to stay at home and just poke the fire.. To the extent that they are forced to do so is an indication of a power-struggle in society.

Disengagement theory has come in for a good deal of criticism in more recent years, even from a number of orthodox social scientists[2]. Alex Comfort gives a satirical picture of the negative stereotype of the disengaged "old person" in contemporary society:

Let us look at the stereotype of the ideal aged person as past folklore presents it. He or she is white haired, inactive, and unemployed, making no demands on anyone, least of all the family, docile in putting up with the loneliness, conscious of every type of boredom, and able to live on a pittance. He or she, although not demented, which would be a nuisance to other people, is slightly deficient in intellect, and tiresome to talk to, because folklore says that old people are weak in the head, asexual, because old people are incapable of sexual activity, and it is unseemly if they are not. He or she is unemployable, because old age is second childhood and everyone knows that the old make a mess of simple work. Some credit points can be gained by visiting or being nice to a few of these subhuman individuals, but most of them prefer their own company and the company of other aged unfortunates. Their main occupations are religion, grumbling, reminiscing and attending the funerals of friends. If sick, they need not, and should not, be actively treated, and are best stored in institutions where they can be supervised by bossy matrons who keep them clean, silent and out of sight. A few, who are amusing or active, are kept by society as pets. The rest are displaying unpardonable bad manners by continuing to live, and even on occasion of complaining of their treatment, when society has declared them unpeople and their patriotic duty is to lie down and die[3]

Although the above is deliberately exaggerated, it contains many important truths. Some people, even at quite an advanced age, are highly reluctant to be regarded as "elderly or old" because of the negative connotations of such terms, and some research studies have confirmed this[4] People don't like the label "old", particularly when it is applied to a woman – to call someone of either sex an "old woman" is definitely derogatory! Thus a woman over the age of 60 may be perceived not just as someone who happens to have been born before a certain date, but as an "old person", and therefore presumed to be a bit slow in the uptake, and to possess the various other attributes listed by Comfort in the quoted passage. The idea of such a person having it off in bed, particularly with a younger man, and enjoying it, will strike many younger people as grotesque.

Nowadays we hear a lot about the evils of racism and sexism, and there are laws to prevent discrimination on grounds of race and sex. But there are no laws designed to combat ageism.

Love in Later Life in Literature.

The fact that older people have erotic needs, fall in love, and form new relationships, has been almost wholly ignored in literature throughout the ages. We have to go as far back as Aristophanes' *Ecclesiazusae* to get an honest recognition of the fact that many women have a need for erotic love when they are old, just as they have when they are young. The theme is that the women of Athens have taken over the government, and recognizing the need of elderly women for a sex-life, they enact a law that no young man can have his girl-friend without first giving sexual service to any elderly woman fancying him. Three women, identified as "hags", lust after the same young man, and prevent him keeping tryst with his girl-friend. The play is a brutal satire, and most feminists would find it grossly offensive, but it recognizes the facts of life which were acknowledged in ancient Greece, as they are not acknowledged today – that age makes very little difference to a woman's sexual appetites.

A more humane view in classical literature is taken by such writers as the Greek lyric poet Philodemus; he celebrates the erotic capacity of older women:

> *Charito is more than sixty*
> *Yet her hair is still a dense forest*
> *No brassiere holds up the marble cones*

Of her high-pointed breasts.
Her unwrinkled flesh exhales ambrosia
And myriads of teasing charms.
Lovers, if you do not run from hot desire,
Enjoy Charito
And forget her many decades[5].

But here the poet Philodemus displays a macho male's attitude to female sexuality, in that he praises Charito simply because she *resembles* a younger woman, but he misses the point about what constitutes attractiveness in older women. An older woman can still be attractive when she no longer has high-pointed breasts and an unwrinkled skin. The attractiveness of an older person lies in the character of the face, which can still be striking and charming despite the many wrinkles, and an attractive personality is conveyed by the whole body. For instance, Bertrand Russell was far better looking and attractive in old age than he was as a young man.

The idea that later life should be a time of renunciation of sexuality finds some expression in the ancient world, but their attitudes were ambiguous. In *The Republic* of Plato we read:

I was once present when someone was asking the poet Sophocles about sex, and whether he was still able to make love to a woman; to which he replied, "Don't talk about that; I have left it behind me and escaped from the madness and slavery of passion." A good reply I thought then, and still do. For in old age you become quite free of passions of this sort and they leave you in peace.[6]

But as both Sophocles and Plato were reputed to have adolescent boys as their bedroom playmates in their peaceful old age, their retirement from heterosexual hurly-burly may not mean what many people think of as "Platonic" love.

In the Christian tradition, Chaucer, following Boccaccio, generally adheres to the convention of condemning erotic love in later life. We have already mentioned his tale of the "old" knight January marrying May, and being made a fool of accordingly, but Chaucer speaks up for the rights of older women through the Wife of Bath who, with her youthful beauty gone, still boldly declares that she will welcome a sixth husband. Shakespeare's generally negative attitude has been mentioned, as has that of Congreve. Charles Dickens gives several examples. We can sympathise with poor Madelene Bray, in *Nicholas Nickleby*, whose selfish father wishes to marry her to the horrible old Arthur Gride, and this "selling off" of young women to elderly bachelors was probably a not uncommon practice in Victorian England. But when Dickens introduces the case of an older woman contemplating a love-affair he becomes positively vitriolic. He admitted representing his own mother as Mrs Nickleby, and presents a cruel picture of her believing that the man next door has fallen in love with her, while it is evident that the poor man is hopelessly insane, and the methods of his wooing are utterly grotesque. Whether Mrs Dickens ever did have such a passion in later life is unknown, but Charles Dickens uses the theme for a general satire on older women.

Among the more modern writers who have written a good deal about the theme of love, sex and power, such as Colette, Thomas Hardy, Henry James, D.H. Lawrence, Somerset Maugham, Proust, Shaw, – their novels and plays largely ignore the fact that people can fall in love in later life, and that such love can be as great and as meaningful as love in youth and middle-age. This is curious, as in their own lives many of them encountered examples of newly-formed love-relationships among people of quite advanced age. There are signs that this neglect is changing. Several writers have discussed the extent to which older figures are given prominence in modern fiction, and where the validity of erotic interest and erotic need in such elders can be admitted, and reflects the changing balance of power between the generations. Bashevis Singer, the famous Yiddish writer, deals with "old love" in his stories, and he holds that, "In love, as in other matters, the young are just beginners". This emphasis seems related to the fact that, being Jewish, he is not writing in the Western Christian tradition which has perpetuated certain assumptions about the elderly which are not really true. The Christian tradition has been to suppress elderly people, to deny them their full status of personhood, and to try to get them to spend their last years abasing themselves before their god and preparing for death, in the words of Prospero:

> And thence retire me to my Milan,
> where Every third thought shall be my grave.

Another modern author in the Jewish tradition who writes realistically about the old is Saul Bellow. In his *Mr Sammler's Planet* he makes Artur Sammler, aged 72, the central character, and he brings out very effectively the association between sexuality and power in a number of places in the book. When the large and aggressive pick-pocket corners and menaces Mr Sammler, he expresses his threat and power simply by forcing him to look at his huge erect penis, a gesture that is a common threat among the males of primate animals. The human animal commonly expresses threat and defiance by saying "fuck you!". When Mr Sammler attempts to lecture to young students and presents a politically unwelcome message, he gets a noisy response and one of them presents their objection to his views and age thus:

> Orwell was a fink. He was a sick counter revolutionary. It's good he died when he did. And what you are saying is shit .... Why do you listen to this effete old shit? What has he got to tell you? His balls are dry. He's dead. He can't come[7].

Thus the young objector to Orwell's ideas, who is presumably a Marxist-Leninist typical of the 1960s, expresses his ageism in sexual terms, wishfully attributing sexual impotence to the elderly Mr Sammler.

Outside the Christian tradition also, we must consider the Japanese writers. Mary Sohngen[8] lists 87 novels published between 1950 and 1975 in America or the U.K. which are written from the perspective of a protagonist over the age of sixty. She comments that among these novels written "During this period when sexual frankness was an accepted element in fiction, only a few includes the sexual activity – or the sexual fantasies – of the protagonist." There are, in fact, seven novels in this category, and two of them are translations from the Japanese. One Japanese novel not mentioned in this list, Sawako Ariyoshi's *The Twilight Years*[9] is of particular interest in that it brings out the extreme dilemma in Japanese culture – the conflict between the Confucian tradition of respect for parents and elders, and the ancient custom of *obasute*, which means literally "discarding granny". It is alleged that in ancient times old people over the age of seventy were taken up the mountains and left there to die, and indeed, there is a mountain on the island of Honshu called Obasute-yama. It is difficult to say how legendary this practice is, but it is commemorated in The Oak Mountain Song.

The Twilight Years was predated by a Japanese short story *The Hateful Age* which, according to Plath[10], has had a significant effect on post-war Japanese attitudes to old people. In this story, the literal practice of *obasute* is not resorted to, but a similar device is employed to get rid of an unwanted grandmother. Here two granddaughters haul the old woman into the country and dump her on the doorstep of a third granddaughter, who by the rules of this ritualized practice, *tarai-ma-washi*, cannot return her. Although influenced by this trend in Japanese literature, *The*

Twilight Years has a curious twist to it at the end. The unwanted old person is a grandfather, Shigezo, a very difficult and selfish old man, who lives with his son and daughter-in-law Akiko. This woman and the old man are the principal characters in the novel; it is upon her that the chief burden of looking after him falls – as well as being exploited by her husband and other members of the family. She openly discusses the doctrine of *obasute* because, of course, such a barbarous old practice can no longer be entertained. Shigezo has always been an egocentric and querulous man, and he is even worse in his frustrated old age; Akiko just has to put up with him, as she puts up with the traditionally boorish treatment from her husband. Towards the end of the book, however, a very curious situation develops; Shigezo's personality appears to change for the better, and in Akiko's presence an unsuspected charm and sensitivity emerges, and it is suggested that he is falling in love with his daughter-in-law. On her part this over-worked and emotionally neglected housewife responds to the horrid old devil, and a curiously tender relationship develops between them. What is it that Ariyoshi is trying to tell us in his novel? That the old are only horrible, selfish old monsters because the society in which they live forces them to be so because it denies them a tolerable role – that the Confucian tradition is mere hypocrisy, and the younger generations would really like to shunt them up The Oak Tree Mountain to die, while they grabbed their goods and the positions they used to occupy?

A further Japanese novel in this genre that should be mentioned is Junichiro Tanizaki's *Diary of a Mad Old Man*[11], in which Utsugi, seventy-seven years old, falls in love with his daughter-in-law. Here the old man is frustrated in his sexuality and becomes more and more kinky in his preoccupation with the woman's feet, but he rightly recognizes that his sexuality is an expression of his desire for life, and keeps him from sinking into apathy and senility.

If we turn back to the literature of the West, one American commentator has observed:

Old age in modern American literature is not the stuff of tragedy. A truly tragic hero must have strength and dignity and purpose. But old age in twentieth century fiction has been denied all of these qualities. When old age appears at all in literary work it is apt to be not tragic, but pathetic. The central theme is the weakness and dependency of old age[12]

But it was mentioned above that there are some signs of modern writers in the Western Christian tradition recognizing that older people do have dignity and purpose, and indeed, erotic needs, although the world of fiction and the world of reality are still far apart. Jewish writers, exemplified above by Bashevis Singer and Saul Bellow, have shown greater appreciation of the facts about old age.

A quite remarkable exception to the writers in the Christian tradition is Graham Greene, who, after a series of gloomy novels in which the Roman Catholic point of view was strongly stressed, went into a period of depression during which he wrote nothing, and then recovered to produce a hilarious novel, *Travels With My Aunt*. This is the tale of a woman in her seventies, who after a lifetime of affairs and actual prostitution, has her sexual appetite unabated, and as part of her generally joyous life-style continues to take new lovers, and ends up happily with one of her old lovers who is even older than she but who shares her immense sexual charm, joy of life, and contempt for bourgeois morality. What happened to Graham Greene in his personal life that caused this volte face is, as yet, unpublished.

We have had one or two black comedies dealing with the horrors of old age in post-war society, such as Muriel Spark's *Momento Mori*, and Kingsley Amis' *Ending Up* and *The Old Devils*, and so far the erotic theme in literature about old people is scarce. Among the signs of a more positive approach that have been developing in the post-war years we have Eudora Welty. Her "Old Mr Marblehall"[13] portrays an old man, who married for the first time at the age of sixty, regarded by his neighbours as having one foot in the grave, and having one son born of this elderly marriage. But having built up the picture of an old man living sedately with his dull wife and solitary offspring, the story then reveals that Mr Marblehall has, in fact, two wives with a son by each and manages successfully to lead a double-life, chuckling to himself at his own duplicity and maintained virility, so that secretly he manages to retain the habits of his randy youth, despite the stifling atmosphere of a life-denying society that would relegate him to the scrap-heap of the old and used-up if they could.

When V.S. Pritchett began to get quite old himself, he took to writing about older people defying the stereotype of "the old" that society projects on them, and using the theme of the erotic impulse to remind people that they should try to live in the present, and not in the past when they were much more physically vigorous. He has his character Mr Dawson, who is aged seventy and a widower, (in "The Spree"[14]) say, "I must not fall into *that trap:* old people live in the past. And I am not old! Old I am not!".

Mr Dawson meets a widow, and at first he regards her simply in terms of the conventional "old woman", noting the signs of age on her face, but later he realizes that his real need is "not for a face or even a voice or even for love, but for a body." The idea that some people of this age who are deprived need sex, as an immediate concern, more than companionship or love, may seem shocking to those in our society who are conditioned to accept the Darby and Joan stereotype of elderly people, as in the mawkish poem of Robert Burns:

> *John Anderson, my jo, John,*
> *We clamb the hill taegither;*
> *And monie a canty day, John,*
> *We've had wi' ane anither:*
> *Now we maun totter down, John,*
> *But hand in hand we'll go,*
> *And sleep taegither at the foot,*
> *John Anderson, my jo.*

Of course old people want love, companionship and secure relationships, but so do people of all ages. The very young may play around for a while, but their sexual experimentation normally leads to genuine love-relationships of some permanence. There is no reason at all why people in later life who find themselves single should be any different, except that they have often been through experimentation in their younger years and are more aware of what they want. Men are less likely in their later years, to have the compulsive need to prove themselves and, in the words of the old song, "To fuck all the women and fight all the men." But are some of them seeking sex just to prove to themselves that they are not senile? Well, that may be true of certain cases for both sexes, but if so it is better that they should try to keep the life force alive, rather than following the model advanced by Robert Burns. Take heed of Dylan Thomas:

> *Do not go gently into that good night,*
> *Old age should burn and rave at close of day;*
> *Rage, rage against the dying of the light.*

There are, alas, all too many pensioners who are prepared to "go gently into that good night", living on a pittance and prepared to give up their personhood in every way. No political party will espouse their cause, except in so far as those out-of-office will use their plight as a stick to beat those now-in-office. First they must change the image of older people.

Apart from Eudora Welty and V.S. Pritchett, we have Bernard Malamud's *In Retirement*, William Trevor's *The General's Day*, and John Cheever's *The World of Apples*, all works of fiction discussed by Celeste Loughman who says:

> In their most limited sense, these stories extend to the elderly the liberal sexual attitudes which other segments of the population have been experiencing. More than that, they challenge long-standing myths which have become codified into rigid social norms that have effectively severed old age from other stages of life. As behavioral science confirms, the persistence of the sexual impulse gives evidence that life is a continuum and that behavior tolerated in the young should not be censured in the old[15].

At least a beginning has been made among writers who are breaking with tradition.

The Image of the Elderly on TV

In the 1970s there were various studies both in the U.S.A. and the U.K. which showed that older people were almost invisible on T.V. When they did appear in programmes it was either in the role of dear old sweeties mouthing platitudes in the background, or horrible old figures of fun acting as an occasional foil for the real characters, whose young lives were the focus of interest. Pressure was brought to bear on T.V. companies by groups like the Grey Panthers who insisted that people over the age of sixty did exist in society, and that their lives were as important as those of younger people. With something like 18% of the population being in this age group, this is something of an understatement! Changes began to occur in the programmes showing that it pays to kick up a fuss, and of course TV companies are sensitive to the complaints of consumers of the products they advertise. A study in Cambridge in the U.K. in 1984[16] showed what changes had occurred by then.

What is of special interest is the degree to which programmes included or excluded elderly people. While all types of programme had instances of elderly people being totally absent, their absence was particularly noticeable in some. But older people appeared more frequently in programmes concerned with the news, current affairs and documentaries, and this was to be expected, as many prominent people in the world are elderly; in fact if you are rich enough and powerful enough it doesn't seem to matter what age you are . As noted earlier, something like 18% of the population of the U.K. can now be classed as elderly, a fair presentation of group or crowd scenes would naturally present them in this proportion, or a little less, as perhaps they are less publically visible. They were found to be roughly 10%-20% present in scenes where groups were shown.

One striking feature of this inquiry relates to the sex of the elderly figures shown. Although there are a lot more women among the elderly population, they were grossly under-represented in the TV programmes, and they were seldom in central roles. As for the class structure, over four fifths of those appearing belonged to the managerial and professional classes. This bias wasn't so pronounced in fictional programmes where older working-class women had some significant role in popular soap operas such as Coronation Street. Taking into account both the sex and class distortions of the general presentations, the authors of the research say:

> The result can only be called a caricature of the real social world of the British elderly.... an important reason why the elderly as we know them are negligible in television appearance is because the successful elderly people who do figure there are not regarded as elderly in society. Thus, even when they are themselves biologically elderly, politicians and leaders do not represent the elderly as a social category[17]

An attempt was made to rate the elderly shown in the programmes on various characteristics, such as "wise/foolish", "active/passive", "fit/infirm", and one characteristic that proved to be very obviously different from the other was "sexually active/inactive", because it simply didn't apply in so many cases and so wasn't rateable. This was even true bearing in mind that it was not the run-of-the-mill elderly who are shown on TV, but a rather superior class of people, and overwhelmingly male.

Things have improved on TV over the last five years or so, partly due to agitation from pressure groups but also because many older people who have a bit of money have changed in their attitude: they are no longer prepared to hoard it for the sake of their descendants. Knowing that they can't take it with them, they are now beginning to spend it in order to live more comfortable lives, thus forming an important new market. Purchasing power counts with the TV advertisers, and they have been making some attempt to woo the older viewer. Thus we have been getting programmes like "Tea and Sympathy" where three sets of lovers appear – young, middle-aged, and elderly. No longer is Granny deemed fit for the loony-bin if she is considering whether to have it off with her latest beau. Granny has a little bit of money, yes – but now she is prepared to spend that money, so she cannot be safely ignored.

The Image of the Old in Popular Humour.

Jokes are a sensitive barometer of how people feel about things, hence the popularity of sex jokes and lavatory humour in the aftermath of Victorian prudishness, and of black political jokes in repressive regimes. There have been a number of studies of how the perceived ridiculousness and nastiness of growing old is reflected in popular humour. One review of jokes about old people revealed that over half of them showed a highly negative attitude, and *ageing women* were the especial butt of aggressive humour[18]. Another review[19] compared jokes concerning the elderly with those about children, and found that whereas most of the jokes about children were appreciative, viewing them in a positive if "quaint" light, most of the jokes about old people were definitely derogatory, ridiculing them because they were supposed to get stupider as they aged, and mocking their physical decay and the decline of their sexual powers. A few jokes were more complex, however, turning upon those who denigrate the elderly because their turn to be ridiculous would be coming in the course of time. Some jokes affirmed that some old people have a lot more life in them than is generally supposed, old men being shown as being absurd whatever they do, as they are seen either as sexless wrecks or over-sexed lechers.

There are two theories of the meaning and function of jokes that are worth considering, the disparagement theory and the incongruity model. It is easy to interpret jokes about old people in terms of disparagement theory, but unlike racist and sexist jokes, the younger people who make them know that they themselves will eventually be joining the group that is the butt of their humour. There is no way in which they can avoid taking on all the alleged characteristics of the stigmatized group except by dying young.

In the incongruity model, there is a necessary paradox to be perceived – that the crowing young man taking pride in his strength and virility, will one day have to accept the decline that is in store for him. This is the riddle of the Sphinx that was posed to Oedipus – he who walks on two legs at noon, will hobble along on three in the evening – i.e. he will have to use a walking stick when he's old..

That ageist jokes are particularly derogatory of women, is an example of the tragedy of the macho male's approach to sex, the knowledge that whoever he loves for her blooming, youthful charm, will be taken from him inevitably when she changes with age into someone he can't approach in the same way.

In studying popular humour, we may look at greeting cards of various sorts. Birthday-card humour displays examples of aggressive ageism, often combined with sexism. There is, of course, the traditional mother-in-law joke; this aged female figure, ugly, stupid and domineering, has no counterpart in a father-in-law figure.

A. I've formed quite an attachment for my mother-in-law.
B. How strange!
A. Yes, it fits over her mouth.

The older woman represents what the young wife will become in the course of years. Birthday cards are particularly significant, as they remind people of the passing years and of the spectre of old age that looms ahead. Those designed to be sent to older relatives are typically sentimental and cheerful, reassuring the recipients that they don't look their age; it is those designed to be sent to contemporaries that contain crude jokes about the coming of old age with all its supposed horrors.

In summary, we may say that all ageist jokes display just what racist and sexist jokes display – fear. The "Rastus" jokes against negroes, display the fear of the dominant white man that those he exploits will rise up against him; sexist jokes against women betoken that the exploited female will likewise emancipate herself from his dominance, and ageist jokes show a fear that old people will no longer accept their status of pathetic old fuddy duddies, fit only to poke the fire and look after the grandchildren. The revolution is already under way, and anarchists are at the fore-front of it![20]

Chapter 2: Notes

1. See E. Cumming & H.W. Henry, *Growing Old: The Process of Disengagement*. Basic Books, 1961. Also: E. Cumming, "Further thoughts on the theory of disengagement". *International Social Science Journal*, 1963, 15, 377-393.
2. See J. Dowd, "Aging as exchange: a preface to theory" *Journal of Gerontology* 1975, 30, 584-594.
3. Alex Comfort, *A Good Age* Pan Books, 1989.
4. R.A. Ward, *The Aging Experience* Harper & Row, 1954.
5. W. Barnstone, *Greek Lyric Poetry* Bantam Books, 1962.
6. Plato *The Republic*. Penguin Books, 1955.
7. Saul Bellow, *Mr Sammler's Planet*. Viking, 1970.
8. Mary Sohngen "The experience of old age as depicted in contemporary novels". *The Gerontologist*, 1977, 17, 70-78.
9. Sawako Ariyoshi, *The Twilight Years* (Trans. M. Tahara) Peter Owen, 1984.
10. D. Plath, "Japan: the after years" In D.O. Cowgill & D. Hughes (eds.) *Aging and Modernization*. Appleton-Century-Crofts, 1972.
11. Junichiro Tanizaki, *Diary of a Mad Old Man*. (Trans. Howar Hibbett). Alfred. A. Knopf, 1965.
12. D. Fisher, *Growing Old in America*. Oxford University Press, 1977.
13. Eudora Welty, *A Curtain of Green*. Doubleday, 1941.
14. V.S. Pritchett, *The Camberwell Beauty*. Random House, 1974.
15. Celeste Loughman, "Eros and the elderly: a literary review". *The Gerontologist*, 1983, 20, 182-187.
16. J. Lambert, P. Laslett & H. Clay, *The Image of the Elderly on T.V.*, University of the Third Age in Cambridge, 1984.
17. Ibid.
18. E. Palmore, "Attitudes towards aging as shown by humour. *The Gerontologist,* 1971, 11, 181-186.
19. J. Richman, "The foolishness and wisdom of age: attitudes toward the elderly as reflected in jokes". *The Gerontologist*, 1977, 17, 210-219.
20. About the most revolutionary book published which attacks the public stereotype of ageing, and urges older people to rise up on their own behalf over a broad front, is Alex Comfort's last anarchist publication, *A Good Age* (op. cit. Introduction).

CHAPTER 3

The Attitudes of Conservative Doctors and other Professionals

People are likely to come in contact with health-care and other types of professional workers increasingly as they age because of their failing vigour and, alas, their increasing poverty if they are wholly or largely dependent of the State pension. Individual doctors in general practice vary enormously in their competence in dealing with older people, and in their attitudes towards them. In competence, because their professional practice has been so largely with the young and middle-aged in the past that they have little experience of or knowledge of the sort of disabilities that occur in later life. It is only more recently that they have had a large number of elderly people among their patients. As to their attitudes, the conservatism of the medical profession is well-known. Almost every progressive innovation in medicine has been in the teeth of opposition from the profession as a whole. They originally opposed the proper training and registration of midwives; they opposed the introduction of anaesthetics in surgery – arguing that it was good for patients to suffer pain; at the beginning of this century they opposed the giving of contraceptive advice to working-class women at a time when birth-control was being widely if secretly practiced by the middle-class; they opposed the spread of sexual enlightenment by teaching utter rubbish about the supposedly dreadful effects of such normal practices as masturbation[1].

Those individual doctors who have been far-seeing and enlightened have always had a hard job promoting their reforms against opposition and the simple inertia of their colleagues. Medical students have traditionally been recruited from rather reactionary strata of society. Things are changing now, but the rate of change is slow. There are two main reasons why many doctors oppose progressive change: the first is trade-union opposition to developments which give related professions such as nursing and midwifery, clinical psychology, and physiotherapy, more power. The medical establishment wish to retain power in their own hands and be in control of all other professions who work in health-care, even when the other professionals are far more knowledgeable and skilful in certain areas. The second reason is sheer emotional irrationality. Young medical students tend to be horribly embarrassed in dealing with elderly people, particularly when it concerns anything like sex. They would rather regard older people as "old dears" who can be fobbed off with palliative medicines, whatever is wrong with them, until they obligingly kick the bucket. Medical student humour is full of crude ageist jokes.

Among those responsible for the training of medical students are a few brave and enlightened doctors who are aware that maintaining the health of patients in later life depends on more than just dishing out tranquillizers and sleeping tablets. They realize that the maintenance of health at all ages is bound up with living a fulfilled emotional and sexual life. All too often medical textbooks appear to inculcate in students an assumption that they can safely ignore the sexual needs of older people. Thus in *Medicine in Old Age*[2] there are 22 articles which appear to take this assumption for granted when sexuality is relevant to what is being discussed: for example, the possible side effects of impotence attendant on the prescription of certain drugs for the elderly is not even mentioned; thus older men are being rendered impotent by the drugs their doctors prescribe for them. Hormone replacement therapy for women is mentioned, but not for the most obvious use that some post-menopausal women require it – the maintenance of vaginal lubrication and the general enjoyment of their sexiness. These omissions are quite shocking, and it is difficult to believe that that it is entirely accidental that some medical writers seek to keep students in ignorance. Medical students' negative assumptions about the elderly may be reinforced by such textbooks.

There have been attempts to modify the attitudes of medical students towards the elderly but they don't appear to have been very effective[3]. More successful have been the attempts to modify students' attitudes towards sexuality in general. Dr Elizabeth Stanley describes a programme that she and her colleagues initiated at St George's Hospital in London[4]. Basically the programme consisted of showing the students a series of 17 short films in six sessions, dealing very explicitly with various sexual situations, and discussing the students' own reactions in seminars. The sessions referred to: (i) ordinary heterosexual relations; (ii) masturbation; (iii) homosexuality; (iv) situations involving lovemaking in pregnancy, with physical handicap, and between "older" people; (v) body-communication with autistic children; (vi) sex therapy. According to the later seminar discussions and a questionnaire, the students' attitudes appeared to have been modified in a positive direction, and it emerged that:

> Encouraging numbers felt that their attitudes had changed towards greater acceptance and understanding about each topic in the questionnaire, particularly in relation to sexuality in the elderly and physically handicapped[5].

We are told that in the love-making scene between the couple representing the "elderly", the man was aged 63 and the woman 50! This is hardly what most people would consider to be "elderly". The man was 13 years older than the woman. and one wonders what the students' reactions would have been if the couple had both been in their 70s, or the woman had been considerably older than the man. Perhaps the intention was to let the students down lightly without too great a transgression of traditional prejudices.

If a pretty young woman goes to her doctor to discuss her sex-life she will be unlikely, nowadays, to meet with other than a sympathetic hearing, and some effort will be made to help her. Indeed, if the doctor is a man, she may meet with quite enthusiastic interest! But if the woman is in her seventies the doctor's reaction may be very different if she goes on precisely the same mission. "What's the randy old bag bothering me about that for? Surely I've got better things to do than to worry about her and her toy-boy. She should realize that she ought to be well past it!" Have patients equal rights? Well, only if they are prepared to stand up for them. Elsewhere[6] I have recounted how a friend of mine in his sixties went to his doctor about a urinary problem, and on his inquiry whether the proposed treatment would affect his sexual potency, was met with amused incredulity. The doctor tried to imply that he really shouldn't be concerned with such things "at his age".

Quite recently I conducted a survey of all the medical schools in the U.K. inquiring what sort of attention they give to teaching medical students about the needs of elderly people[7]. I got quite a good response, and it is evident that a number of medical schools are beginning to introduce more teaching of social gerontology, that is, about ageing from a social as well as a sheerly medical standpoint. From one such enlightened school the professor makes the point that their object is not to train "embryonic consultant geriatricians", but to equip the students:

> with the skills and attitudes necessary to care for elderly people. One particular lecture is given by an elderly lady who describes the sexual attitudes as they were when she was a girl and goes on to describe how her own sexuality (and that of her husband) evolved over the years. This lecture provides very pertinent insights for the young students[8].

The great wealth of information that modern research has given the medical profession about the disease processes in later life has presented a certain dilemma in teaching: how to balance the direction of students' studies between the diagnostic aspects of medicine and the treatment of various pathological conditions that afflict a small minority of older people, and a necessary appreciation of the nature of the physical and emotional well-being of the normal majority who need some attention from doctors in their role of counsellors and specialist advisors. In the past, geriatric medicine over-emphasised the former aspect of the doctor's role. A consultant geriatrician responded to my survey by writing:

> The essence as I see it of teaching geriatric medicine is to emphasise not only diagnostic and investigative aspects of disease but to emphasise the emotional aspect and the physical and mental consequences of disabling disease in old age.... Another major component of the undergraduate course is trying to teach the skills of communicating with elderly people who have got problems with communication and this surely has a lesson for dealing with older people in general[9].

One consequence of teaching students about the most serious pathological conditions that occur in old age, necessary though it is, is that they may get a biased view and fail to appreciate how basically healthy and potentially vigorous most elderly people are, *given the right social and personal environment*. Another Professor of Geriatric Medicine mentions this, and how he tries to overcome such bias. He writes:

> The clinical practice of our department is that we take responsibility for the frailest and most disabled of the elderly patients in the hospital, deliberately seeking out those with the most complex multiple disability....There is, of course, a real risk that

this will give a distorted view of normal ageing, emphasising all the dreadful things that can happen, and leading the student to forget the fact that most elderly people are relatively untroubled by such problems. This is an important issue which we address with our students in my introductory seminar[10].

I have tried to pick out the most positive replies that I received in my survey to emphasise that there are far-seeing and even radical medical doctors in influential positions who are trying to steer the profession along progressive lines. If people meet with obstruction and less than adequate consideration from the G.P. they happen to have registered with, they should certainly make their dissatisfaction known and insist on a transfer until they get an adequately competent and properly sympathetic doctor. Times are changing, and it is up to us to promote the change.

Other Health-Care Professionals

If medical doctors are a very mixed bunch, what about the other health-care professionals? The nursing profession has gone through enormous changes in the post-war years and more changes are on the way. It used to be that the majority of hospital patients were in the care of women known as "dragons" – the ward sisters – who were the terror of the young nurses. As for the patients, the most important thing was that their beds should be tidy and that their bowel motions were regular – never mind whether they were in pain or not. Do I exaggerate? Some may object to my using such strong language when there were many excellent and humane women working as ward sisters and doing their best to improve the system. But for the earlier part of this century I don't exaggerate if we consider the run-of-the-mill sisters (and, of course, matrons). The history of the nursing profession, from Florence Nightingale onwards, is scarred by the whole oppression of women and its consequences in Victorian England, and furthermore, the horrible slaughter of a whole generation of young men in the 1914-18 war left a generation of single women, many of whom were understandably embittered. A lot of these women went into the nursing profession in the 1920s and materially affected its tradition. There used to be a cynical saying that "God gets the women whom men didn't want – or they find careers in nursing." The more humane nurses often got married and left the profession as soon as they could, and the higher up the nursing hierarchy one went, so grimmer "dragons" were to be encountered in the bastions of power. Although the nursing profession has nowadays changed very substantially for the better, there are still some of the old guard in positions of petty authority, and unhappily they find appointments controlling geriatric wards and as matrons of old people's homes. Consider the following scene in a modern hospital, as described by Alison Norman:

> An old lady is wheeled from the ward bathroom to her bed area on a hoist, the seat of which is about four feet from the ground. She is inadequately covered and her bare buttocks hang through the commode-type seat so that her anus is exposed to view. Her bottom has not been dried and looks sore. She is weeping as she is wheeled along. While this scene is taking pace, a clinical tutor from the associated Teaching Hospital is visiting the ward. She smiles as she greets the student nurses who are transporting the old lady in this fashion[11].

The author of the above, Alison Norman, is not an irresponsible young radical, but a very experienced authority on ageing, who used to be the Deputy Director of the Centre for Policy on Ageing. She goes on to quote another document:

> If patients are to be parts of a well-oiled machine, they cannot be seen as people – as individuals clinging to the vestiges of personality, choice, dignity and independence – as individuals who have lived long and full lives and have now lost the place in the community which gave them a role and identity – as individuals who are now living in "social death". So, the pain is buried in activity and routine; the patients are railroaded into passive conformity; and the message transmitted all too easily becomes "We are caring for your body" but "You as a person do not really exist."[12]

I am reminded of our old comrade Matt Kavanagh, dying in a hospital in the Forest of Dean, while his friends were endeavouring to arrange for his transfer to London, and the ward sister officiously arranging for a catholic priest to visit him. According to Matt, "He hung over me like a bleedin' black vulture, trying to get at me soul – and there's me having to fight the bugger off!"

As with the medical profession, some of the nurses are in revolt against the old authoritarian Florence Nightingale tradition, and there has been some lively controversy in their paper, *The Nursing Times*. The expression of sexuality by the inmates of an old people's home or a hospital may cause great embarrassment to some of the nursing staff. Thus Emily Griffiths, a staff nurse, relates how, when seeking to comfort an elderly man, she held his hand and asked if she could do anything for him; he replied by suggesting that she should get into bed with him, a suggestion she was not inclined to accept. She goes on to observe that:

> There are two main reasons why sexuality in the elderly is diffi-
> cult to discuss. First, nurses historically have not been trained to
> cope with sexuality. Their sexuality is 'suppressed and repressed',
> with the aim of 'purity' and 'asexuality', and they suffer from sex-
> ism and stereotyping at work. But if nurses are not aware of
> their own attitudes, beliefs and values, they will not be able to
> help others[13]

The second reason for embarrassment in discussing the expression of sexuality among older people that she gives relates to the ageism of a youth-oriented society, making it difficult for older people to verbalize the nature of their emotional feelings for fear of being seen as depraved and lecherous. She states that while there is a considerable literature on counselling following medical and surgical interventions, she couldn't find any referring to patients' need for sexual expression, only some on "inappropriate sexual behaviour in residential homes". While no-one would suggest that it's part of a nurse's job to get into bed with the elderly people she looks after, if she is sufficiently well balanced, she should be able to handle the situation tactfully and without making a fuss.

It may be questioned whether the taboo on facing the reality of sexuality among older people is now as strong as it used to be. One very simple reason why sexual activity in old people's homes etc. is discouraged, is that it is administratively inconvenient. It would suit the administrators far better if both men and women, when they reached a certain age, were simply un-sexed and there would be an end to it. They would be much, much more docile, like castrated cattle.

Dominique Wright, a Staff Nurse, observes that it's now generally accepted that sexual activity is "important for emotional and general well-being", and she goes on to say that although the nursing and social work press are just beginning to question traditional attitudes to sexuality in the elderly, "Sexuality is not even acknowledged or catered for." How far that is still true in the nursing profession is questionable. She goes on to state:

The literature suggests that health workers need to look at their own sexuality and also gain some understanding of the subject. Perhaps we then can cater for the client's needs. I think that this is particularly important for nurses. We claim to be concerned with the whole individual and yet we ignore an essential part of that individual's life. Some of the issues in this article have great implications for health educators and workers. The elderly often get a rough deal; perhaps we can start improving the situation by acknowledging their sexuality[14]

Reviewing these various publications, it seems that the nursing profession is in a state of transition, and what evidence we have about the current attitudes of young and not so young people towards the emotional lives of the elderly, and how far sexuality needs to be expressed, is somewhat contradictory. What needs to be fully realized is the extent to which the issue of power is bound up with sexuality. Bossy matrons don't just object to their elderly "charges" getting into bed together because they aren't getting it themselves, but because they are seeking to rob them of their full adult status in order to exert power over them more easily.

Social Workers

We have discussed the attitudes of the doctors and nurses towards elderly people in general, now what about the social workers? This profession has quite a lot to do with those who need help because of the infirmities that come with age – particularly when poverty becomes automatically linked with age. Social workers come in all shapes and sizes, and in recruiting them there has been a muddled attempt to attract people who are themselves suffering from various disabilities. If we look at the booklet giving details of the training courses for social workers run at all the university and polytechnic departments, we get the following statements that are repeated again and again:

> Applications from candidates with a disability is (*sic*) encouraged
> – In situations where several candidates are seen as equal, the
> course favours the more disadvantaged candidates – People with
> a limited recent education are encouraged to apply – those with
> family commitments or disabilities are encouraged[15].

Now it is estimable to provide work for people who have failed in other jobs because of their disabilities, and who are pretty well unemployable elsewhere, but the zeitgeist of social work goes further than that. It is held that people make better social workers if they are variously impaired because they will have more sympathy and empathy with their clients. But there is not one scrap of evidence to indicate that this is so. It might be argued that people who are in special need would benefit more from the services of those who were able-bodied and without significant psychological disturbance. Someone who has a problem of mobility is not necessarily best aided by a social worker who cannot climb stairs because he or she is in a wheel-chair; a client who is in trouble because of his schizophrenic attacks, is not necessarily best served by a schizophrenic social worker; a girl living in the bizarre world of anorexia nervosa is not necessarily helped most by an anorexic social worker, and a compulsive kleptomaniac may not get the best help from a professional person who frequently pinches things from shops.

The world of social work is rather bizarre. From time to time we read of awful scandals where wretched children have been repeatedly mistreated and eventually murdered by psychopathic adults, while well-meaning social workers have hovered in the background, giving excuses for their non-intrusion. Also, social workers seem repeatedly to blunder, taking children from perfectly ordinary families into care because they (the social workers) suffer from fantasies about "satanic abuse"[16]. Many people are very puzzled why this should happen with such lamentable frequency, but it doesn't surprise me at all because I've come in personal contact, over a period of some years, with the training of social workers. I know only too well what a wide spectrum of psychological disorder is covered by this term "disability" which is so prized in the recruitment of social workers. It seems to me inevitable that if people are deliberately chosen because of their inadequacy, the mess they have made of their own lives, and their failure to meet the ordinary standards of employability, they are likely to make a hash of any job they do, and their clients will suffer.

But to get back to the question of social workers' role in helping elderly people who are in trouble, and understanding their needs, let us consult some actual data, and, of course, try to identify some of the more progressive trends in social work. I have tried to get in contact with the more realistic and competent social workers who are well aware of the troubles of their profession. Some social workers are specially concerned with the problems of elderly people, and they have their own informal association[17].

The thesis of this book is that elderly people should demand their rights and change their image in society. They are entitled to expect services from professional workers like anybody else, and that such services should not only ensure minimal standards of nutrition, health, and adequate housing, but contribute to their general emotional well-being and enjoyment of life *according to their own personal standards.* This doesn't meet with unqualified approval from all social workers, many of whom just aren't interested in what they see as the boring problems of old age. Let us see what their primary interests are. When discussing the training provided for the nursing and medical professions, we quoted from some progressive individuals who were concerned that serious and deliberate attention should be given to students' attitudes to older people in general, and to their emotional and sexual lives. There's not much evidence that such concern is shown in relation to trainee social workers. In *Paper 30*, under the heading of "The Values of Social Work", it is stated that qualifying social workers must be able to:

demonstrate an awareness of both individual and institutional racism and ways to combat both through anti-racist practice. develop an understanding of gender issues and demonstrate anti-sexism in social work practice[18]

While it is entirely laudable that awareness of the issues of *racism* and *sexism* should be part of the training of social workers, it is significant that *ageism* is just not mentioned at all. Certain prejudices against older people, particularly in relation to the conduct of residential homes, has long been a feature of the care of the elderly. Professor Stout[19] points out that, "Attitudes towards the elderly, of both the population as a whole and of some members of the health professions are sometimes unhelpful and negative". I would also quote Alison Norman[20] again, who says that "some social workers felt that elderly people, as compared with children, had had their lives and have no future contribution to make to society, so why bother about them?" No doubt this question comes in for a good deal of discussion in some training courses, but it does not feature prominently in the journals associated with the social work profession. Looking back in the file of *Community Care*, the social workers' main journal, references to older people principally concern issues of housing, dementia, hypothermia, home care services, and other bread and butter issues. There is little evidence that it is recognized that "man cannot live by bread alone", or that social workers are trying to live up to the avowed aim of contributing to the quality of the majority of their clients' lives, irrespective of their age. There might be more debate about the emotional needs of older people in the social work journals. There are exceptions to the general neglect. Dr Skinner, in the above-mentioned journal, makes quite a forceful plea for the sexual needs of older people to be considered by social workers and the staff of residential homes, and argues that:

> It is important to be aware that a satisfactory sexual relationship is important for most people's well being at any age. In the elderly the increased need for love, self-esteem and for close human contact give sexuality an enhanced value....Professional staff need to be aware of compounding the problem through projecting their own taboos by, for instance, discouraging developing liaisons[21].

But Dr Skinner is not a social worker; he is a psychologist.

The social workers' special interest group in the elderly, referred to above, might be expected to explore the relevant issues in greater depth than the profession as a whole. They were given a talk on *Sexuality in Later Life* by Dr Mary Davies; this appears to have been a somewhat unusual occurence. It should be noted that Dr Davies, like Dr Skinner, is not a social worker but a psychologist. In a personal communication, a very senior social worker associated with their Special Interest Group on Ageing, writes:

> I recall no mention of the sexual lives of older people on my professional course, and my colleagues in my area office ... report the same of their training courses ..... The absence of expertise is reflected in books on social work with older people. We rely possibly on organisations like Relate and their counselling skills. We are only just beginning to tackle principles and procedures in Social Service Departments about sexual abuse of older people. The residential sector of social work may have more to say about sexual expression than fieldworkers like myself. Maybe I am being unfair on the social work profession, and it would be gratifying to learn through your reseach whether there are social workers having lively discussions. Let's hope that in the assessment of older people's needs with the community care plans of 1991 we are required to tackle their sexual needs[22].

* * *

Perhaps it may be thought that in a book such as this too much is being made of the services provided by the State for elderly people through its agents. Should we not look more to self-help rather than depending on the State? Such a view overlooks the fact that it is these very people who, through a lifetime of work, have provided the wherewithal for doctors, nurses etc. to be trained, and that they have already paid their wages whether or not they accept their services! The astonishing fact is that many elderly people don't claim the benefits that are properly due to them. According to the Department of Social Security, in 1985 900,000 people failed to claim the benefits to which they were entitled, and this applied particularly to Supplementary Benefit – 79% of elderly people who were entitled to it failed to claim it! Is this due to irrational pride, to apathetic acceptance of poverty, or mainly to a strong revulsion from having any truck with bureacracy? We should encourage people to stand up and yell for the right to enjoy what is, in fact, their own, and to resist being put down by the ageist assumptions of our time.

Chapter 3: Notes

1. For a discussion of the absurd medical pronouncements about masturbation in the nineteenth century, see M. Hollender, "The medical profession and sex in 1900." *American Journal of Obstetrics and Gynecology*, 1970, 108, 139.

2. British Medical Association, *Medicine in Old Age*. B.M.A. 1985.

3. C.W. Smith & J.R. Wattis, "Medical students' attitudes to old people and career preference: the case of Nottingham Medical School." *Medical Education*, 1989, 23, 81-85.

4. Elizabeth Stanley, "An introduction to sexuality in the medical curriculum." *Medical Education*, 1978, 12, 441-445.

5. Ibid.

6. H.B. Gibson, "Do G.P.s take the sexuality of older people seriously? *The Raven*, 1991, 4, 251-255.

7. H.B. Gibson, *The Emotional and Sexual Lives of Older People: A Manual for Professionals*. Chapman & Hall, 1991.

8. Professor A. Personal communication to the author.

9. Dr B. Personal communication to the author.

10. Professor C. Personal communication to the author.

11. Alison Norman, *Aspects of Ageing: A Discussion Document*. Centre for Policy on Ageing, 1987.

12. Ibid.

13. Emily Griffiths, "No sex please, we're over 60." *Nursing Times*, 1988, 84, 34-35.

14. Dominique Wright, "Sex and the elderly". *Nursing Mirror*, 1985, 161, 18-19.

15. *Qualifying education and training in social work: college based routes*. CCETSW Leaflet 9.2. November 1989.

16. See Donald Rooum, (op. cit. Introduction).

17. British Association of Social Workers – Special Interest Group on Ageing.

18. *Paper 20: Requirements and regulations for the Diploma in Social Work*. Central Council for Education and Training in Social Work, 1989.

19. Robert W. Stout, "Teaching gerontology and geriatric medicine". *Age and Ageing*, 14 (Suppl.) 1-36.

20. Alison Norman, op. cit.

21. R. Skinner, "Young at heart." *Community Care*, 11th Feb. 24-25.

22. Neil McKenzie, personal communication to the author.

The Self-Image of Older People:
The Legacy of the Repressive Past

How do people who are over the age of retirement regard themselves? This has been the subject of a number of interesting inquiries, the results of which may come as a surprise to many younger people. Dr Paul Thompson[1] and his colleagues carried out a long series of interviews with men and women over the age of sixty and published the results under the title of *I Don't Feel Old*[1], which is what most people of the older generation say nowadays. They would probably not have said this a few decades ago, for there has been a definite change in attitudes in the post-war era. When addressing people over the age of 60 years, we should be careful as to how we refer to their age-status. A surprisingly large number of such people will be slightly offended if they are referred to as "elderly" or "old". The unthinking reference to "An old lady like you...." may be displeasing to a woman in her seventies who doesn't regard herself as "an old lady". Russell Ward[2] interviewed 320 men and women aged in their 60s, 70s and 80s, and asked them how they would classify themselves with respect to their age-status. While 172 referred to themselves as "elderly" or "old", 148 saw themselves as "young" or "middle-aged". How such a question is posed makes quite a lot of difference, but it was clear that some even in the oldest age group didn't regard themselves as being "old". Ward tried to find out why people would see themselves as being in one or the other category, because it may seem to many younger people that someone in their 80s who doesn't see himself as "old" is just plain silly. However, it's not as simple as that. The main determinants of older people's perception of their age-status are health and productive activity. Thus sickly men or women in their early 60s, who have retired from work and have no particular occupation, may regard themselves as "elderly or old", whereas healthy people in their 80s who are still busily occupied, either gainfully or voluntarily, may still see themselves as no more than "middle-aged", and may indeed have long ago given up bothering about their age.

When they get to a certain age, quite a number of people realize that the whole business of age-status is rather an illusion. All their lives they may have expected to be "old" when they reached a certain date on the calendar, but when they reached it they didn't feel any different. They realized that they were still "young" in their inner being and perception of themselves. Occasionally a man in his 80s may say that when he attends gatherings of retired people, some much younger than himself, he looks around the grey heads and wrinkled faces, and thinks to himself "Poor old fellows – I'm glad I'm not like them!" Simone de Beauvoir observed that "old people are also mirrors for one another, mirrors in which they do not care to see themselves – the marks of old age they behold vex them"[3] The viewer sees the externals, and because of his long conditioning by society's stereotypes of age, he can't realize that many of these people feel just like he does in their inner selves.

Poor Old Me?

Age is no excuse for being less efficient and energetic in trying to solve problems, and facing up to one's responsibilities, although a lot of people take refuge in playing "poor old me". There is even a recognized condition known as "pseudo-dementia", in which people act daft as though they really did suffer from some such a horrible condition as Altzheimer brain damage, and expect other people to take care of them. We should be charitable to such people (we may end up like that ourselves!) for they have generally been the subject of some very tragic circumstances, but we should be aware of the reality of the situation. With care, they can be brought back to normality. There is a tendency for older people to be treated differently from younger people because; (a) it is thought that the poor old things can't be expected to feel and behave as ordinary human beings; (b) that in certain areas of life their needs are less important than those of younger people. It is up to all of us who are "getting on in life" to fight these assumptions *tooth and nail*. And younger people too should fight ageist assumptions no less vigorously, for one day they too will be old, and inherit a world which is governed by the traditions of the past.

There is a story of a man aged 103 who went to his doctor complaining that his right knee was rather stiff, and demanding treatment. The doctor saw that he was not seriously incapacitated and, being unable to suggest any useful treatment, took refuge in saying "Well, that knee is 103 years old, so I don't see you have much to complain of." The patient replied, "Well the left knee is also 103 years old and it's all right – so what are you going to do about the right one?"

The fact that someone looks "old" and is indeed a very senior citizen according to the date of birth, doesn't mean that he or she is in any way different, intellectually, emotionally or socially, from a younger person. Much depends upon the individual. Although we have just discussed how health determines, to some extent, people's perception of themselves with respect to age-status, health is a relative matter. One can be sickly at any age, yet still feel and act vigorously intellectually and emotionally. In a very large research study conducted by Edward Brecher[5], among people of quite advanced years a remarkably large proportion of both men and women reported being sexually active, and with a high enjoyment of sex – despite being in only fair or poor health, and despite the seven adverse health factors that were reviewed. The fact that some people in the last decades of their life take up totally new careers, develop fresh and absorbing interests, fall in love, and give other signs of that intangible quality of a "positive mental attitude" is evidence that the *potential* for living life to the full need not evaporate with age. How is it then, that quite a fair number are such dreary old wrecks, taking refuge in pomposity, the "poor old me" game, and other irritating ploys?

The Question of Work in Later Life

Let us consider what Pablo Casals, the great Spanish musician, said when interviewed at the age of ninety-three:

> On my last birthday I was ninety-three years old. That is not young of course .... But age is a relative matter. If you continue to work and to absorb the beauty of the world about you, you find that age does not necessarily mean getting old. At least, not in the ordinary sense. I feel many things more intensely than before, and for me life grows more fascinating....
>
> Work helps prevent one from getting old. I, for one, cannot dream of retiring. Not now or ever. Retire, the word is alien and the idea inconceivable to me. My work is my life. I cannot think

of one without the other. To 'retire' means to me to begin to die. The man who works and is never bored is never old. Work and interest in worthwhile things are the best remedy for age. Each day I am reborn. Each day I must begin again[6].

Well, we can't all be highly gifted men like Casals, but whoever and whatever we are, we can take a leaf out of his book. The institution of "retirement", which was heralded as a great and humane advance in social policy (at least it was better than being shunted into the workhouse) has come to be a very dubious measure. It was enshrined in the great Beveridge Report of the 1940s, as a means of getting rid of people from the work-force at a certain age, and expecting them to live on a pittance for the rest of their lives. Some want to retire from their jobs at an early age – fine, let them do so. Others want to carry on working at their job – and if they are fit for it, why shouldn't they?

Health, Longevity and Sex.

We noted above that health was one of the determinants of whether people felt themselves to be "old" or not, but this needs to be qualified. What is "health"? It might be thought that everyone knows whether they are in good health or not, but that really isn't the case. People may have all sorts of things wrong with them that would be identified by a medical examination, yet if they are living busy, interesting lives, they say they feel all right, and can't be bothered to think much about their health. Conversely, there are people who very preoccupied with their aches and pains, how their bowels are functioning and whether they are getting sufficient vitamins, when there's nothing much wrong with them, other than that they are bored and frustrated. It might be thought that the former type of people who tend to neglect their health wouldn't live as long as those who constantly fussed over it, but as a matter of fact – it's the other way round! There is good scientific evidence showing that subjective health (how people rate themselves) is a better predictor of longevity than objectively determined health[6].

Some people may say that we shouldn't worry so much about longevity – the actual length of time we live – as the quality of life is far more important. I certainly agree with this; most of us would rather drop dead suddenly in the midst of a busy, happy life, than slowly peter out, wracked with increasingly severe disabilities. But longevity is associated with *vigour* in later life.

People who are vigorous in old age tend to live a long time. Let us look at the age of death of some well-known people: Bernard Shaw (94), Eamon de Valera (93), P.G. Wodehouse (94), Fred Streeter (98), Hewlett Johnson (92), Bernard Leach (92), Winston Churchill (91), Gordon Craig (94), Norman Angell (95), Gilbert Murray (91), J.P. Powis (91), Bertrand Russell (98), Sidney Webb (97), Mannie Shinwell (100). I quote these as a few examples; I could extend the list much further, and add some female names e.g. Grandma Moses (101), because they've come from a research project I've been doing, but the point is not just that they all lived into their nineties, but that they continued to be *active* in their various spheres of life practically until the day of their death. My research followed a lead I got from elsewhere, and we can make several statements: (i) People who marry live longer than those who never marry; (ii) men who are bereaved have a greatly increased risk of death the first year after their wife dies, but bereaved women aren't similarly affected; (iii) men who re-*marry* after the age of sixty tend to live longer than men who don't. There are various interpretations that one can put on these facts; it does look as though love and sex in later life, prolongs life, just as interesting work appears to, but the issues aren't clear cut. If we look at another research which was carried out at Duke University[7] in Northern Carolina, the picture begins to become clearer.

In this research, they studied a population of men and women, median age 70 years, for a period of 25 years. Here are some of the findings concerning marriage and sex as they relate to longevity. Frequency of intercourse was a significant predictor of longevity for men. For women, this was not necessarily as important, but past enjoyment of intercourse was a significant, moderately strong predictor of longevity. Health was the strongest predictor of longevity, and it may be noted that the health-measure was *self-rated* health, which may be a better predictor of longevity than objectively rated health, as was noted earlier, although objective examination by a doctor may discover conditions unknown to the patient.

Can it be argued, then, that the act of sexual intercourse – and enjoying it – does something to our bodies so that we are more vigorous and live longer? Our old friend Wilhelm Reich certainly believed that and elaborated a rather fantastic theory about "orgone energy" to substantiate his belief. Before we examine the theory further, let us consider just what has been the traditional belief about vigour in old age and longevity.

The Search for the Elixir of Youth.

The search for the secret of longevity, the "elixir of youth" is a very old one, and we haven't space properly to consider its history here. There has always been a belief that longevity was in some way connected with sexuality, and many of the ancient nostrums that were supposed to promote longevity contained material from the sexual organs of animals. One of the first attempts to rejuvenate men in terms of modern medicine was that of Charles Brown-Sequard who injected himself with testicular material from various animals and claimed that it had produced in him renewed vigour and enjoyment of life. This was in 1889 when he was 72 years of age; he died five years later. Experiments with various species with the transplantation of the testes of young animals into the bodies of senile animals, convinced some scientists that this would eventually lead to a practical means by which human life could be prolonged. Such work is principally associated with the names of Steinach and Voronoff: Voronoff implanted the testes of monkeys in elderly men and claimed that this did indeed rejuvenate them, but as the experiments weren't properly controlled, there was no evidence that it had any effect on their life-span. From what we now know about organ implantation, and the actual effects of the injection of testosterone, the male hormone, it is plain that Voronoff's experiments could have had no relevant physiological effect on his patients, but their status was probably improved by the placebo effect.

Later research into longevity has turned away from such crude physiological experimentation to anthropological and sociological inquiries. This doesn't mean that physiological research isn't relevant and important in the study of ageing; unquestionably it is, and the steady accumulation of physiological knowledge about ageing processes will certainly pay off in the future, but no quick solutions are to be expected. Later research, for a time, turned to studying the life-style and health of human populations in natural settings. From this all sorts of ideas about diet and life-style excited researchers right up into the 1970s, when it became plain that the data on which they were based were pretty useless. The populations in various parts of the world – notably Ecuador, Kashmir and Abkhazia, had been claiming to be very long lived and misleading the researchers. It is difficult to conduct such inquiries in places where the registration of births a long time ago was not very accurate, and where the people themselves, proud of their reputation, have a motive for exaggerating their age.

Various later researchers have thrown doubt on the validity of the supposed findings, and have produced evidence that the supposedly long-lived Ecuadorians actually have a life expectancy less than that of the population of the U.S.A.[8]

There's no evidence that any special diet or way of life is particularly productive of a long life as far as a whole population is concerned. Obviously, if populations are living in conditions of mal-nutrition and disease, as in many parts of the Third World, the life expectancy will be low, but what we are concerned with in such cases is early, and preventable death.

Sexual Co-habitation and Longevity

It has been shown that there's some evidence that widowers who re-marry will have longer lives than those who don't, but this doesn't necessarily mean that there is any magic virtue in the sexual relationship. We may go no further than considering a common-sense explanation for this fact. Loneliness, depression and idleness are potential killers because they predispose people to lose the will to live. In an emotional state of misery people tend to indulge too heavily in drinking, eating an inadequate or badly balanced diet, smoking excessively, and taking all sorts of dangerous risks with their health. If they are badly housed without adequate warmth in winter, they are less likely to bother to do anything effective about it. They are specially vulnerable. Deaths by suicide form a significant percentage that steadily mounts with age, reaching 27 per 100,000 for males of 85 years and over in England and Wales in 1988. This is almost certainly an under-estimate, as doctors are reluctant to attribute a death to suicide if another cause is plausible. However, this is only the visible tip of the iceberg of men who are despairing of life and longing for death.

It may be asked why men who have remarried are slightly longer-lived than those who have simply stayed married, and pre-deceased their wives. Although the married state is certainly a protective condition for most men, and enables them to live longer, it is no guarantee of continued appetite for life. The widowed men who re-marry later are likely to be people who show some determination to make the best of the remainder of their lives. All that's been said earlier applies also to women, but to a lesser degree. Women in general aren't so badly affected by bereavement as men, at least in terms of their raised mortality; married women live only slightly longer than those who are single, widowed or divorced, and their suicide rate in later life is about a half to a third of that of men of equivalent age.

Is there, then, hard evidence that sexual activity in later life actually increases longevity? Does love-making do something to our bodies so that we're more vigorous, and less subject to the ravages of time? Possibly it does, but we can't prove it. However, even if it *shortened* our lives, I expect most people worth knowing wouldn't be deterred from their love-lives by such a calculating decision to be ascetic and abstinent. Fortunately there's no such negative evidence!

> *Abstinence sows sand all over*
> *The ruddy limbs and flaming hair,*
> *But desire gratified*
> *Plants fruits of life and beauty there.*

Good old Billy Blake!

Conclusion

This chapter is principally concerned with how people see themselves, and it's been shown that it is the self-image, especially with regard to health, which largely determines how vigorous they will be in later life even though they may have all sorts of things wrong with them which are the natural consequence of the body wearing out. We are all going to die some day, and we hope the end will be sudden, for we also hope that we'll continue to be pretty active, independent and enjoying life. The image of us having all sorts of things wrong with us may sound depressing, but the fact is that most of us *at any age* have a lot wrong with us we don't know about, but if such malfunctions don't inhibit our general functioning and enjoyment of life, why worry?

The question of sexuality is important, because most people need to be conscious of their masculinity or femininity, whether they are eight or eighty. A man of eighty may regard his fucking days as over (although a lot don't) but he is no less of a man, and as fully conscious of his masculinity as he ever was, and the same goes for women as concerns their feminity.

Someone may now ask "What about those people who are naturally homosexual?" Well, a homosexual man is still a *man* whatever age he is. It is a mistake to regard the minority whose erotic preferences are towards their own sex, as being neither men nor women, and the mistake derives from the huge folk-lore about "nancy-boys" etc., etc. Unfortunately, this folk-lore has influenced the self-image of many homosexual people, so that a homosexual man in his sixties may come to regard himself as an "ageing queen" and adopt all the music-hall affectations of that stereotype. In this context, some people may also be puzzled by the instances of transvestites, cross-gender switching, hermaphrodites etc., but these need hardly concern us here as such individuals are such an infinitesimally small minority – although played-up no end by the sensational media.

Finally, what about those women who have been heterosexual all their lives, married, and who have perhaps raised families, who take up a lesbian life-style in later life, partly because of the great shortage of men in the later decades? In general, they are no less feminine, although living sexually with another woman; but again, fashion may influence them to dress in a special way.

But to come back to the population in general. What they are up against as they age is the stereotype of the "aged" that is wished on them by tradition. If they accept that stereotype, which embodies all the myths that were described in Table 1 in Chapter 1, and really begin to feel and behave like that as they age, and consequently they will be pushed into a powerless, workless, sexless, underpaid underclass, nonentities whom many people hope will hurry up and die. If, however, they are sufficiently independent-minded they will resist any such change in themselves, and encourage others in their age-group to do the same. Solidarity, comrades, solidarity!

Chapter 4: Notes

1. P. Thompson, C. Itzin & M. Abendstern, *I Don't feel Old*. Oxford University Press, 1990.
2. R.A. Ward, *The Aging Experience*. Harper & Row, 1954.
3. Simone de Beauvoir, *Old Age,*. Penguin Books, 1972.
4. E.M. Brecher, *Love, Sex, and Aging: A Consumer Union Report*. Little, Brown & Co., 1984.
5. A.E. Khan (ed.) *Joys and Sorrows: Reflections by Pablo Casals*. Simon & Schuster, 1970.
6. J.M. Mossey & E. Shapiro, "Self-rated health: a predictor of mortality among the ageed". *American Journal of Public Health*, 1982, 72, 800-808.
7. E.B. Palmore, "Prediction of the longevity differences: a 25-year follow-up." *The Gerontologist*, 1982, 22, 513-518.
8. R.B. Mazzess & R.W. Matheson, "Lack of unusual longevity in Villacomba, Ecuador." *Human Biology*, 1982, 54, 517-524.

CHAPTER 5

Towards a New Concept of Sexuality

What do we mean by sexuality? This is by no means as simple a question as it seems. Writers like Freud caused a furore in their day by attributing sexuality to the motivation and behaviour of infants, and interpreting much adult behaviour in terms of "sex", and Wilhelm Reich likewise caused puzzlement and stirred up hostility by going even further in trying to trace the connection of sexuality with social and political power. Yet stepping our perspective back a bit historically, Ernest Gellner, a modern philosopher, demonstrates that much of what Freud wrote was by no means original, but was expressed in the philosophy of Friedrich Nietzsche:

> one finds in Nietzsche's work a rather general entity, the Will to Power, whereas Freudian theory is preoccupied with sexuality. It is not entirely clear whether the Nietzschean Will to Power is simply a generic name for all striving, like Schopenhauer's Will, or whether it is a little more specific. Admittedly, Freudian sexuality also often looks like something much broader than sexuality in any normal sense. The libido seems fairly free-floating. It lusts after What it May Concern, rather than some circumscribed object. Nevertheless, there seems to be a contrast between the two thinkers at this point, and Freud does at least seem to be much more specific[1].

We shall certainly not get much enlightenment from the study of such a turgid and bombastic writer as Nietzsche, but it is important to realize that Wilhelm Reich was not taking such a very original step forward from his master, Freud, when he proposed the thesis that the expression of sexuality was essentially bound up with the aspiration to achieve legitimate power, and one way of denying people their full power was to suppress their sexuality.

What does Sexuality mean to us in our Later Decades of Life?

There are many problems associated with the continuance of sexual activity in later life, or its renewal after a period of celibacy following widowhood. Why shouldn't older people resign themselves to living celibate lives in some circumstances? If they're married, or living in a long-term relationship, they could carry on for the sake of companionship, but not worry if the physical aspect of the relationship comes to a complete end. If they find themselves rendered single, should they aspire to form new sexual relationships? After all, it's admitted that the physiological drive for sex dies down in intensity with age, at least with men, and it may seem that there is little point in stoking, rather than damping down, a furnace that can lead to all sorts of social inconveniences.

It's entirely understandable if some people see the situation in these terms, especially if they have a vested interest in "castrating" the older generation. We discussed earlier why people in administrative positions, such as the matrons of old people's homes, would find it more convenient if all their charges were docile, sex-less beings. Similarly, some middle-aged children may resent signs of continued sexuality in their parents for reasons of mercenary expectation of inheritance, or sheer emotional jealousy. They may find it difficult to understand just what is being pioneered in this and similar books and journals. Is it right, they may ask, for organizations such as Age Concern to encourage the grandparent generation to expect to lead a full sex-life? Will the randy old beasts never give up?

To answer this question, it's necessary to explain a concept of sexuality that applies in later life, and is rather different from that which characterizes the younger years of adulthood. Most older people may take some time fully to realize the physiological and psycho-social changes that will take place over perhaps the last 30 years of their lives, and if they hope to recapture precisely the same sort of sexual satisfactions that they had in youth and middle-age, they will be disappointed. Yet sexuality in later life can be fulfilling and of great importance to many people, although some people at all ages seem to lead well-adjusted a-sexual lives. It takes all sorts to make a world!

We discussed in the last chapter how throughout life most people need to regard themselves positively with regard to their feminine or masculine sexuality. This is generally a deep psychological need, and denial of it may lead to depression and preternatural ageing. As people age, they're subject to subtle psycho-social changes, as well as physiological changes. If a man tries to cling to a macho image of being a frequent and efficient phallic performer in his later decades of life, he might as well try to compete in the athletic contests he used to go in for half a century before. With unrealistic expectations he'll be heading for trouble, and may perhaps suffer from performance anxiety, so that eventually he comes to regard himself as "impotent", and withdraws from love-making altogether. But with a more sophisticated understanding of the expression of emotional feeling in physical terms, he may enjoy a lifetime of rewarding love-making in which phallic performance, appropriate to his age, need not play such a major part. With a woman, the problem is different, but there's no reason why she should ever lose her sense of femininity, or to cease to be attractive to the right person despite her growing wrinkles.

For many people, "sex" means copulation with the goal of the male orgasm, conceived of as the ejaculation of semen. Although most intercourse is engaged in not for procreation but for recreation, this goal tends to be greatly over-emphasised. However, this traditional view of sex has been becoming modified in more recent years, partly due to the feminist movement, but also due to the work of sex-researchers and therapists. When sex therapists have asked people what they really want of sex, the answer appears to be pleasure, satisfaction, psychological contentment, a sense of self-worth and a celebration of their love for their partner. These are the real goals of love-making, rather than the limited traditional goal. Seen in these terms, the validity of homosexual love-making is apparent. If the lover is of the same sex, so what? Love is being expressed.

It has been pointed out[2] that the language which many people use in referring to sexual activity emphasises the "getting to" rather than the "experiencing of" a pleasureable activity. The terms "foreplay" and "afterplay" emphasise that there's a "big event", a goal which has to be reached, and all else is subsidiary. Some feminists have complained angrily of the male definition of sex - that it lasts "until *he* comes" - and then it is all over! The emphasis on peno-vaginal intercourse culminating in male orgasm as being the essential and defining characteristic of lovemaking, is regarded by many feminists such as Hite[3] as merely fulfilling a macho male need to boost their egos. Her investigations of female sexuality showed that many women's feelings of fulfilment in sex depended on a far broader range of activities involving intimate sexual techniques. Some women have never experienced orgasm in intercourse, but experience it regularly or occasionally through manual or oral contacts in lovemaking.

One of the greatest insights that an ageing man can achieve is to realize that his masculinity doesn't depend wholly on his phallic prowess, and that an experienced lover will be able to give and receive sensual pleasure and emotional satisfaction through the wide range of lovemaking techniques that are generally known by sex-therapists as "pleasuring", which we shall discuss later. The misconception that "foreplay" is something that the man does to the woman just in order to get her ready for him to penetrate her needs correction. Rather, the more satisfactory aim is to achieve a level of physical and emotional interaction between the couple. Whether or not this involves peno-vaginal intercourse later on, is another matter. Some quite young couples go in for what they call "non-penetrative sex". There are no *musts* in love-making. Some couples achieve their sexual pleasure without actual copulation, and where the man doesn't respond with full erection, genital intercourse is perfectly feasible with a flaccid penis, provided that the woman is in a sufficient state of sexual arousal to accept it vaginally.

We mentioned earlier on that older men should ask themselves "What do I need sex *for* - is it a compulsive effort to demonstrate to myself and others that I am not yet a worn out 'old man'"? Many people use the rituals of love-making for purposes that are basically a-sexual, and this is pretty pointless. Some researchers have found that even among younger people, many women enjoy the total experience involving all sorts of caressing. We may call this "fore-play", but it doesn't necessarily come before anything. Younger men tend to say that the act of intercourse is more important to them, but this may reflect a strong psychological as well as a physical need, and it may not apply to older lovers if they are happy about their male identity and feel no need to prove themselves.

Women sometimes get a raw deal if their male partner, finding that his phallic performance is declining with age, withdraws entirely from all sexual encounters out of pride. She's still as ready for love-making in all its aspects as she ever was, but she may have to endure a total deprivation for many years because of her husband's "impotence". This cruel deprivation may be inter-preted by her as being all her fault, attributing it to her ageing appearance, and some men who will give this as a reason for their withdrawal from sexual relations. Bernard Starr refers to "the tyranny that the male erection holds over the potential for intimacy, physical stimulation, and sexual pleasuring", and goes on to write:

> Pleasuring refers to any sexual experience that feels good. With pleasuring there is no one act that measures or validates the success of the experience. There are just different events, intercourse and orgasm being just two, neither of which is necessary or essential for a pleasurable experience. Within the context of the pleasuring definition of sexuality, adults of all ages are on an equal par. Frequency and degree of sexual pleasure are limited only by interest, desire, and imagination. While the frequency of different acts may vary, (e.g some may have more frequent intercourse than others), the potential for pleasuring is open to couples with whatever frequency is desired, regardless of erectile response or age. From this point of view, some of those who seek and achieve intercourse could conceivably experience less pleasure and, therefore, less sexuality than those open to and skillful at a variety of forms of sexual pleasuring[4].

Full credit must be given to the original studies of Masters and Johnson who, in their therapy for younger couples, popularized the idea of "pleasuring" without intercourse as a valuable aspect of love-making that may, or may not, lead to intercourse.

Should there be Sex Education for Older People?

Some older people, particularly men, may regard the idea that they may be in need of sex education with indignant horror. "What *me*? who's had more pussy than you've had hot dinners! Get away with you!" may be the reaction. But whatever constituted "having pussy" in their younger years may have little relevance to their later experience.

Information about sex in later life may come as a great liberating influence for many men and women, relieving them of guilt and pressure to perform to an unrealistic standard. It's liberating to realize that there are enormous natural variations between people, and between couples, as to their expression of sexuality, as became apparent from the early studies of Kinsey and his colleagues. Older people need liberating from all sorts of irrational taboos: for instance, a woman in her seventies may begin to suffer from arthritis, which makes it painful to spread her legs in the face-to-face position of intercourse that she has enjoyed all her adult life. She may never have copulated in any other position, and indeed, have regarded other positions (if she has heard of them!) as being somewhat "perverse" and not within the province of decent sexual relations. Her husband may be too shy to urge her to vary their usual practice, regretfully accepting that they must abandon all intercourse because of her arthritis.

It needs to be pointed out to such a couple that their difficulty may be solved by using other techniques, such as the man lying behind his partner, and that such a position is neither "perverse" nor uncommon. Similarly, all sorts of sexual techniques that are described in modern sex-instruction books, that younger people practise for fun and for variety, are very suitable for older people whose minor disabilities make the continuance of their usual forms of love-making more difficult. Here we come to one of the great difficulties in imparting knowledge to many, although not to all, older people. Some may say, in effect, "But surely such antics are only for the young - it would be unseemly for us to behave in such a way, or even to discuss it together!"

The Shyness of the Elderly of the Present Generation

The following incident illustrates a very real problem. There is organization, the University of the Third Age, which now has autonomous branches in quite a number of countries, and caters for the interests and activities of people who are mainly, although not entirely, over the age of retirement. At a recent international conference convened by a branch in a university city, there were various eminent speakers lecturing on topics of special interest to older people. It was announced that many of these speakers had books of their authorship on display and available at a nearby bookshop, and attenders at the conference were invited to go there, browse, and buy them. These books attracted some attention, and there was quite a sale of them, with the exception of one author. This was Alex Comfort, whose talk was much appreciated, but the only two books of his the bookshop displayed were *The Joy of Sex* and *More Joy of Sex*, which were left severely alone. These two books, although they contain some sensible facts and advice on ageing, are lavishly and quite tastefully illustrated with drawings of young and comely men and women making love in a great variety of ways, and this was enough to put off older people from buying them openly, or to be seen reading them in a bookshop. I know a woman in her 60s who has one of them in a brown envelope in her desk, whereas a younger woman might display it openly on her bookshelf, without giving much thought to its presence. The older generation still have a struggle to get their legitimate aspirations accepted by society.

In a booklet published by Age Concern[5] there is a humourous cartoon showing the notice board of an old people's home in which various activities are advertised - knitting, recipe swop, bingo, pottery, and kamasutra. While each activity attracts a few ticks, it is the kamasutra class that attracts a whole cluster of ticks, and an old lady is shown adding hers.. This may represent the wish, rather than the reality, but it would be interesting to see how such an offer was received if it were really included among the other voluntary classes and activities in such a home.

It's difficult, therefore, to get the older generation to buy, borrow or read books of sex instruction, even though they may be quite educated people. They are embarrassed to be reading such books *at their age*, and pretend they don't need them.. In the 1920s and 1930s when such books came widely on the market, they were often sold in "rubber goods" shops, along with condoms, douches and Dameroids, or sold in back-street bookshops which dealt in surreptitious pornography, and they may still retain this image in the minds of many older people. The fact that Comfort's sex books are now attractively presented and sold openly in respectable bookshops is all to the good, but their bold appeal to the young, makes older people shy of reading them.

Comfort's re-issued paperback *A Good Age* is well illustrated with pictures of older people, but none of them are making love. It has a good section on sexuality in ageing. Age Concern have published the booklet mentioned above *Living, Loving and Ageing*[5] which is directed to the reading public and is mainly about the sex lives of older people, offering much sensible advice. One criticism may be made of this book: it unintentionally presents a rather negative image of sexuality in later life because it highlights all the things that *can* go wrong, failing to indicate just how rare these morbid conditions are. The senior author, Wendy Greengross, is a medical doctor with a reputation for helping the handicapped, so it is natural that her experience of older people will be atypical. Since doctors are primarily concerned with the sick and the handicapped, they have less experience with the healthy old who are the majority and have less need of their services. Their book deals in considerable detail with various conditions such as amputated penises, faecal incontinence, implanted catheters, colostomy, prolapsed vaginas and suchlike, and some readers will find these passages grisly reading.

Obviously the unfortunate people who have such conditions need help and advice regarding their sex-lives, but discussion in a doctor's surgery, or with a visiting health-care professional, would seem to be the appropriate situation, rather than in a popular paperback. Some people who are approaching later life may get the impression from this book that all these disabilities may be in store for them and their partners as they age, and reflect that they would rather give up lovemaking altogether than have to cope with the handicaps attendant on faecal incontinence, an implanted catheter, a prolapsed vagina etc.! It must be empha- sised that the main impediments to a satisfying love life in our later years are not *physical* at all, but *psychological*, the product of the negative image that sex in later life has in most people's perception of it, and that what is chiefly needed is to improve this image.

There is a dearth of good books dealing with sex in later life, and directed to the reading public of average intelligence. But however good the supply of sex education books suitable for older people is, there's the problem that it's not always easy to get people in the older generation to read them. They would like the information, but are reluctant to get it from a book.

The giving of advice about sexual matters to people of more limited education often falls to doctors and other health-care work- ers, and Hawton makes the point that:

> It is unwise to assume that a couple have a sophisticated know- ledge of sexuality; very often a couple who give this impression will be unwilling to admit to areas of ignorance, or be unaware of their blindspots. A fairly didactic educational session, in which pictures are used, is helpful. This session should be tailored to needs and problems, as well as the educational level, of the individual couple[6].

The paradox here is that more educated and superficially sophis- ticated people may be the ones more prone to pretend to a greater knowledge of sexuality than they possess, whereas less educated and simpler men and women may freely admit to the extent of their ignorance. There is, of course, a class-difference in sexual vocabulary. Most people's sexual vocabulary may be very differ- ent from that of the professional person giving the advice. While less educated people may not know the meaning of words such as "vulva" or "fellatio" - or have an inaccurate knowledge of what they mean - professional people may not know the vernacular terms commonly used by their clients, and which vary from district to district. A further difficulty arises because some vernacular terms serve the double function of referring to sexual organs and practices, and of being coarse swear-words. A working-class man or woman, particularly of the older generation, might be very shocked to hear a professional person using such vernacular terms, and it requires some experience and tact in acquiring a vocabulary of words that are "acceptable" demotic terms that refer to sexual parts and functions in a particular part of the country. Felstein[7] gives an intelligent discussion of this question and provides a glossary of various demotic sexual terms. The best we can do in this book is to refer readers to the list of publications given in Appendix 1.

In summary, we may say that if people can only take a more advanced and sophisticated view of sexuality, they'll appreciate that age really doesn't make such a very great difference. We should retain the importance of our sexuality throughout our lives, and relate it to the way we value ourselves, and those around us. A discussion of how sexuality is related to power will be pursued further in Chapter 8.

Chapter 5: Notes

1. E. Gellner, *The Psychoanalytic Movement*. Paladin Books, 1985.

2. See B.W. McCarthy, *What You Don't Know About Male Sexuality*. T.W. Crwell, 1977.

3. S. Hite, *The Hite Report*. Dell, 1976.

4. B.D. Starr, "Sexuality and aging", *Annual Review of Gerontology*, 1985, 5, 97-126.

5. W. Greengross & S. Greengross, *Living, Loving and Ageing*. Age Concern, 1989.

6. K. Hawton, *Sex Therapy: A Practical Guide*. Oxford University Press, 1985.

7. I. Felstein, *Understanding Sexual Medicine*. M.T.P. Press, 1986.

Some Effects of Property-Consciousness and Sexual Jealousy in the Family

T here is a strong connection between property-consciousness and sexuality. In patriarchal forms of society a man *owns* his wife or wives, and the notorious tenth commandment of the Jewish law, which the Christians have taken over, reads, "Thou shalt not covet thy neighbour's house, thy shalt not covet thy neighbour's wife, nor his manservant, nor his maidservant, nor his ox nor his ass, nor anything that is thy neighbour's." In the traditional Judaeo-Christian view, the wife, then, is property ranked higher than the ox or ass, but not as important as the house. A wife is a piece of property that gives many services, sexual service among them, and anyone who makes use of such service, even though he does not damage the property, is guilty of robbery.

An enormous amount has been written about the question of women being the sexual property of men; anthropologists, both serious and amateur, have given us accounts of how the institution of property-ownership, and the institution of marriage varies in a wide variety of simple cultures. While one cannot entirely trust the accuracy of all these studies, the general rule seems to be that the more property-conscious a culture is, the more sexuality is rigidly controlled by law and custom, and women are subject to male domination. The favourite culture held up by many libertarian writers as a shining example of liberal sexual mores is that of the Eskimos, in which guests are treated so hospitably that going to bed with one's hostess is an acceptable custom, and the Eskimos are conspicuous for their dependence on co-operation rather that the ownership of property. As a matter of fact, I believe that there are various Eskimo patterns of culture, and I'm not sure how widespread such a hospitable custom is. Rather, I think that we should depend on our own observations and experience in twentieth-century Britain, which exhibits a very wide variety of mores among different social groups. In general, I think it is a commonsense observation that in property-conscious groups sexual customs appear to be pretty restrictive, whereas in sub-cultures in which people are more given to sharing, and the ownership of property is not very importaant, people are less concerned with controlling one anothers' sex-lives. Margaret Mead observed that, "Jealousy is not a barometer by which depth of love can be read: it merely records the degree of the lover's insecurity"[1]. Property-ownership necessarily implies *security*. The two contrasted views of love are well conveyed in Blake's poem *The Clod and the Pebble*:

> *Love seeketh not itself to please,*
> *Nor for itself hath any care,*
> *But for another gives its ease*
> *And builds a Heaven in Hell's despair ....*

> *Love seeketh only Self to please*
> *To bind another to its delight,*
> *Joys in another's loss of ease*
> *And builds a Hell in Heaven's despite.*

The Clod, who speaks the first verse, is soft and malleable; the Pebble, who speaks the other, is hard and unyielding. Thus does Blake see the two types of love.

In our immediate history we have passed through a period in which not only were women regarded as the property of men, but children were very much the property of their parents. Older people would tend to live rather penurious lives in order to hoard their property for their children to inherit. In return, they expected a much greater degree of obedience from their children, both in youth and middle-age, than is common today. While a certain degree of surreptitious sexual activity on the part of the sons of the family was winked at, provided it never caused scandal, the chastity of daughters was rigidly guarded, and not only because of the unreliability of contraceptive methods. This general repression was not confined to the bourgeoisie alone, but prevailed in all ranks of society. It is natural, therefore, that the whole libertarian movement, in its many different manifestations, has tended to favour Youth against Age. "The Old" were the property-owners, the repressors of the life-seeking aspirations of "The Young".

Now everything is topsy-turvy, for a very strange thing has come about in society, an event that has never happened before in history: the emergence of The Third Age. The whole theory of The Third Age is expounded at length in Peter Laslett's recent book, *A Fresh Map of Life*[2]. Briefly, the thesis depends upon the radical change in the population structure of our society that has taken place during the present century, so that we now have a large body of people over the age of sixty, a phenomenon that has never been witnessed before in history, and this trend is becoming ever more extreme as time goes on. These older people differ from "the old" in previous times, who were an insignificant minority, in a number of important ways. First, they are relatively healthy and active, and second, they have an attitude to property which differs from that of their ancestors. While all too many of them are forced to live on a pittance, and have little property at their disposal, those who do own a bit of capital are prepared to spend it rather than to hoard it. I believe that one can get a car-sticker reading I'M SPENDING MY KIDS' INHERITANCE.

The increase in the number of people in the later decades of life has two main causes. First, the progress of medical science and general public health measures has caused us to live longer; second, the deliberate restriction of the size of families by methods of birth control means that there are proportionately fewer people in the younger age cohorts to replace those who are now aged. In Britain the records indicate that birth control began to be used to a significant degree in the 1870s in middle-class families, and the practice has spread to all classes in the present century, so that we are now a comparatively old community. While the numbers of all those over the age of sixty are expected to rise over the next half-century, the increase will be most marked in the generation over the age of eighty. This section includes those who are the frailest and in most need of medical and social services. How far improvements in public health, and in techniques for treating the disabilities of old age will progress, remains to be seen.

What is the Tension between

the Young and the Old based upon?

Old people don't earn any money and have to be paid a pension. They frequently suffer ills of the flesh so that their crumbling bodies clog up family doctors' waiting rooms and occupy an absurdly high proportion of costly hospital beds. Their younger relatives have better things to do than act as unpaid servants to wrinklies no longer capable of looking after themselves. In short oldies are a damned nuisance all round, and their numbers are increasing at an alarming rate.... There have been suggestions that before too long the state will have to impose a statutory age limit on the right to life. This could involve oldsters receiving on, say, their 75th birthday, a buff OHMS envelope instructing them to attend their local euthanasia depot on the following Wednesday at 2.30 in the afternoon.

So writes Donald Gould in a semi-serious article in the *New Scientist*[3]. This article continues in a light and jocular manner suggesting ways in which the older members of the population could be disposed of for the benefit of the young. It is accompanied by a humourous cartoon to make it clear that it is not to be taken too literally. However, such humour serves to wrap up discussion of an idea that certainly betrays a tension within society, and having been shocked out of our complacency about the inevitability of humane standards in the civilized countries of Europe by one holocaust in the present century by the government of Germany, who planned to murder all the Jews in Europe as a matter of sound, governmental policy, we need to consider that tension seriously. The idea of the changing age-structure leading to a conflict between the generations is by no means new. In his younger days, Peter Medawar[4] referred to the fact that in forty years time we would become the victims of at least a numerical "tyranny of greybeards", but he added "a matter that does not worry me personally since I rather hope to be among their number". However, in a humourous manner he mentioned the possibility of killing people at the age of seventy as a real kindness to them.

These jokey references to a possible state-enforced euthanasia as a means of getting rid of the excess of older people are referred to by Laslett who comments:

But someone not too far away from his seventy-fifth birthday can perhaps be forgiven for asking what would happen if anyone so much as ventured to refer in passing to a holocaust of all black people in conversation with such persons as Medawar and Gould, let alone print and publish remarks to this effect.[5]

All a big joke? But we abhor racist jokes in decent circles precisely because they betray an underlying viciousness of intention. So what about elaborate ageist jokes like those referred to above?

What, then is the basis of the tension within society which is expressed in a semi-serious plan to kill off all people over a certain age? Largely it concerns the ownership of property. In Chapter 2 we considered the Japanese tradition, or myth, of taking old people up a mountain and exposing them there to die, which is celebrated in The Oak Mountain Song. But this custom, if it ever really existed, reflected the natural personal resentment against having to look after a horrible old person making a real nuisance of himself/herself in the family, and depending on the Confucian tradition to justify their senile power. The idea of wiping out all old people *as a class* has wider implications – it is to grab their property.

It may be objected that the majority of old, working-class people don't own much property anyway – so why slaughter them? But to refer to property in this way is monstrous. Who built up and maintained by a life-time of work, all the "fields, factories and workshops" that constitute the wealth of society? Why, those poor scrubbers who are now living, or trying to, on a State pension eked out by a £10 tip at Christmas. They have a greater moral title to be considered the owners of the wealth of society than those who have merely inherited shares. They are as fully entitled to as adeqate an income from the social wealth they have helped to build up as anyone else.

A small, right-wing body in the U.S.A. has as its main political plank the complaint that older people are being far too well treated, and are responsible for an unwarrantedly large share of the public purse, at the expense of the young. This body is known as A.G.E. (Americans for Generational Equity) as described by Minkler[6]. This economically motivated form of ageism has not yet found any expression in an organized form in Britain, but it is a possible development.

The Fable of the Wooden Bowl.

There is a well-known fable concerning "The Wooden Bowl" which makes an important point about the shifting power between generations in families. It is about a three-generation household in which the little son asked his father why Grandad had to eat all his meals out of a wooden bowl. His father replied that it was useless to give the old man anything better, as he would certainly drop and break china. So poor old grandad sat in the chimney corner eating all his meals out of a rough old wooden bowl. Later on, the father heard his little son chipping away in the wood-shed, and went to see what he was doing; he found him with a big block of wood, beginning to fashion it into a bowl. "This will be for you one day, Dad", the little boy told him.

Is your child, if you have one, beginning to make a wooden bowl for you?

Economic and Sexual Tensions

Where older people do have a bit of money put by, or own a house and furniture, conflict within families may develop on a highly personal basis, and economic and sexual considerations may become mixed.

I was recently on a TV show devoted to the question of love and marriage in later life and the joys and problems arising. The producers had got together a large number of older couples who had married or started living together late in life, and some of their children. Among the problems that were aired was the question of children objecting, with very mixed motives, to their parents teaming up with a new partner late in life. One young man in his twenties came with his mother, a widow of about sixty, who wanted to re-marry. He announced that if she did this he would "disown" her. He lived with his mother, and presumably she cooked his meals and washed his clothes; she might have prepared to continue to do this when the new husband moved in; but then young Charlie would no longer be cock of the roost. Whether or not the husband would inherit any significant property if his wife died first, I do not know, but Charlie's outburst indicated motives that were not entirely economic. I am no great devotee of the Freudian concept of the *Oedipus Complex*, but here was a perfect example of young man upset by the idea of his mother "having it off" across the landing while he slept alone with only a masturbatory pillow to comfort him. Maybe I'm wrong in some particulars of this case – I realize that one should not speculate too freely – but it seemed to me that here was the perfect example of the tensions of sex and power, emotional and economic interests, combining.

There were other similar cases given a hearing on this TV show, including that of a woman in her seventies who was literally "kidnapped" ("grannynapped"?) at a registry office by members of her family to prevent her marrying her elderly lover. Later on they eloped and got married in secret – a most romantic tale.

Earlier in this chapter I have referred to the old tradition of authoritarian parents seeking to "own" their children, and run their lives for them, but now in the changed circumstances associated with the emergence of The Third Age, the reverse tendency is coming to the fore. This is not entirely new, and must have existed to some degree in every age. In Joyce Cary's *Herself Surprised* and *To be a Pilgrim* Sarah Mundy is acting as housekeeper and bed-companion to the old solicitor Mr Wilshire, but when he plans to marry her, the family steps in. Sarah Mundy is sent to prison on a trumped-up charge of pilfering, and the old man is brought to heel with the threat of being certified insane by a medical member of the family. The family inheritance is protected.

The Bereavement Ploy.

Bereavement of someone we love is generally a very painful thing, and it has been noted that there is a high death rate among elderly men during the year following the death of their wives. However, proper recovery from bereavement is normal, and where there has been a good and satisfactory relationship between spouses, friends, and parents and children, recovery is quicker and more complete. But when there has been a strained and unhealthy relationship a long-standing neurotic condition may result, a condition that may take many forms. One of these conditions is known as "enshrinement"; the deceased person may be remembered in totally unrealistic terms. However ordinary he or she was, the image preserved is one of perfection, and no rational discussion is possible. Indeed, the dead person may become very useful to the survivor, who uses his or her supposed wishes in the furtherance of their own selfish wants. Just as Hamlet used the alleged perfection of his dead father to slang his mother, and attempt to inhibit her sexually, so children will sometimes use a dead parent to try to control a living one. Butler and Lewis, in their excellent book (see Appendix), give the following common sense advice:

> Children will sometimes try to preserve the memory of their deceased parent (or your former relationship with a divorced spouse) by the process of *enshrinement*.... They maintain a fierce reverence for the past and want to see nothing changed, so they consider any new relationships you enter into an affront to their other parent. You can then find yourself accused of being selfish, insensitive or disloyal; and if they succeed in making you feel guilty, you may be compelled to sever your new relationship. This is a mistake[7].

Butler and Lewis point out that it is sometimes the fault of the parent who originally encouraged an inappropriately close relationship with the child. Well, well, it is never too late to cut the apron-strings, but it's best never to tie them too tightly in the first place. The bereavement ploy may be the expression of a deep-seated emotional tangle – but it can also be a weapon in the armoury of those who have a hard-headed attachment to property.

What do we do about it?

There are two problems here: the wish to acquire the total ownership of the property that belongs to the parent(s), and the emotions of envy and jealousy aroused by the prospect of a parent enjoying a love-life while the child or children are sexually frustrated either by enforced abstinence, or by being trapped within an unsatisfactory relationship. When the two combine, the strong and irrational emotions of the latter fuel the greed of the former.

No doubt anthropologists could instance many different cultural patterns that have arisen to meet this form of tension within families. It hardly needs stating that squabbling among siblings over property can be quite as bitter as that between parents and children. The only anthropological example I can think of is the custom among some gipsy tribes of burning a deceased person's caravan, with all the property it contains, to prevent quarrelling among the relatives. Margaret Mead[8] proposed that there should be two forms of marriage; one form should be sheerly contractual and carry no rights of inheritance. This would be particularly suitable for men and women in later life who wish to live together and have their union officially recognized, but do not wish to provoke conflicts over the inheritance of property. Children might be happier if their parents contracted this form of marriage in later life as it would not threaten their expected inheritance. Such a form of marriage could, of course, be contracted at any age, and it was Margaret Mead's idea that if children were then born, the marriage would be automatically converted to the conventional type. As the institution of marriage becomes less and less important in the society we know today, so people will attach a lesser importance to whether their unions are officially recognized or not. The problem of property remains, and we do not seem to have advanced beyond the theoretical formulation of Proudhon, the theories of Marx about property having been singularly disconfirmed in practice in the Soviet empire and elsewhere!

On the question of sexual envy and jealousy, we must remember that "sexuality" is given quite a wide interpretation in the present book. A middle-aged couple may be quite well suited sexually in the narrow sense, and have no real reason for envy, yet strongly resent the prospect of the single parent of one of them forming a new love-relationship in later life. Here the dynamics of interpersonal power are involved. A single and perhaps lonely parent may be easily "managed", and given the metaphorical wooden bowl, as described earlier; but when such a parent acquires a new partner, there is a mutually protecting *couple* to be reckoned with, and the old parent-child power relationship is re-established.

So what do we do about it? We live in a property-conscious society which is only slowly emerging from the sexual repression of the Victorian age that had so wide an influence in many aspects of human relationships. We should seek to recognize and understand the realities and strive to oppose oppression in all its forms.

Chapter 6: Notes

1. Margaret Mead, cited by J.A. Lee, *Lovestyles*. J.M. Dent, 1976.

2. Peter Laslett, *A Fresh Map of Life*. Weidenfeld & Nicholson, 1989.

3. D. Gould, "Death by decree". *New Scientist*, 1987, 114, 65.

4. P.B. Medawar, *The Uniqueness of the Individual*. Constable, 1946.

5. Peter Laslett, op. cit.

6. M. Minkler, "'Generation equity' and the new victim blaming: an emerging public policy issue." *International Journal of Health Sciences*, 1986, 16, 539-550.

7. R.N. Butler & M.I. Lewis, *Love and Sex After 60*. Harper & Row, 1988.

8. Margaret Mead, "Marriage in two steps." *Redbook*, 1966, July.

The Problems of Retirement

I t is hard to get people to look dispassionately at the question of retirement from work, and the problems that arise from it. When the retirement pension was introduced at the beginning of this century it was hailed as a great and humane social advance. So it was, in comparison with what went before it – the sending to the workhouse people who were so worn out and impoverished by a lifetime of labour that they could no longer support themselves. But the time has come to take a fresh look at what retirement means, and how it affects people's standing in society. We may turn to our old comrade Alex Comfort who generally manages to set the cat among the pigeons and provoke original thought:

> We can only alter the manipulative cost-accountancy concept of retirement, which kicks people out of society when they can't be milked further, by changing society. On the other hand, from the standpoint of self-defence, retirement has to be met, unless you are wholly self-employed, a housewife, an intellectual of a certain kind, or a peasant – these people never retire or don't notice that they have[1]

Referring to retirement as people being "kick(ed) out of society when they can't be milked further", certainly invites one to take a fresh look at what is going on.

At the time of retirement most people are living as man and wife and the amount of time that they spend together greatly increases, although it may not be as great as one of the partners desires. This change in the life-style of one or both partners can have profound and far-reaching effects, and adjustments have to be made comparable to those which are necessary when young people start living together. But when young people adjust to a new way of living, they are generally flexible in their attitudes and adapt relatively easily to a new way of living. They've usually been having sexual relations for some time before sharing a home nowadays, and moving in together makes demands on their willingness to compromise with one another's habits, but the emotional stresses involved don't ordinarily impinge much upon their sexual relations.

At the age of retirement the situation is very different. Older people may be well adapted to sharing a home, but the home may mean something rather different to the two of them. The man may regard it as a comfortable background to his "real" work, that is, his paid occupation, and such part-time activities as home decorating, gardening, and other hobbies are generally simple relaxations which are pleasant, but for which there is never enough time. The female partner, whether or not she has a job, may have comparable leisure-time pursuits which form a background to her more routine and demanding work. She may have come to regard some areas or aspects of the family home as exclusively "her" domain, and the man may have assumed that others are exclusively "his" property. Retirement sometimes results in "trespasses" on the other's domain, a new source of friction. Both partners may have settled into some sort of stable routine in relation to their work, their homes, and their relations with each other. In some circumstances, this may result in a power-struggle in the home.

Assuming that they've continued to engage in lovemaking, their sex-lives too will have settled into some stable routine. Maybe they tend to fall into routine patterns in which they do the same old thing sexually, time after time, year after year, but still, they are having a sex-life. In the same way, most people's work and leisure habits follow some sort of routine, and while they may not provide much excitement, such patterns of habits are generally quite comfortable and peaceful as long as the existing routine is preserved. Upsets may occur with retirement because the whole routine is changed.

Fiction tells us that most men look forward eagerly to retirement to engage more fully in various activities and projects they've never had time for, only to be disappointed when they find that they never get down to doing what they intended to do, and have time on their hands. The reality is somewhat more complex than this, and often relates to the dynamics of their marriage and to issues that we'll discuss later. Social researchers who've studied the question have generally found that for many husbands and wives retirement is a mere bugaboo – distressing in anticipation but enjoyable after it occurs. However, to take an example, in the large study of Edward Brecher's to which we have referred earlier, of the 803 husbands who had retired, 21 per cent said they had mixed or negative feelings about it, and among the 386 retired wives 25 per cent were less than happy about it. That's quite a significant minority.

The Question of Role-adjustment.

Reasonably happy couples may have quite enjoyed one another's company in the limited hours of leisure in the working day, and on the holidays they have taken together, but when retirement comes a new situation of being something like twentyfour hours a day together may arise in some cases, and place a new and intolerable strain on their emotional relationship. A new life is beginning, the life of the "Third Age", and they're apt to look at and re-assess both each other and themselves. Nowadays, a lot of people are taking early retirement, leaving their jobs in their fifties, so the ensuing problems are becoming even more wide-spread, and, as the population structure shifts with ageing, the proportion of the population retiring increases every year.

After retirement, couples who've led a fairly stable and regular sex-life and never bothered to think much about it, now find, perhaps to their own puzzlement and surprise, that sexual conflicts arise just as, perhaps, they occurred in the very early period when they first began to have sex relations. The man's declining potency, the woman's post-menopausal problems (which often have a more psychological than a physical basis), and the changing physical appearance of them both, provide a fertile ground for such conflicts, but it's the difficulty of role re-adjustment after retirement that's often the real energizer of these sexual difficulties, and fuels the bitterness of the conflicts.

Sexual problems arising out of role re-adjustment are often greater for the working-class than for the middle-class. Sex roles in the former were much more rigidly defined 40 years ago when present-day retired couples were young and formed the basis of their marriage. The masculinity of the older working-class man is frequently defined very much by his work-role, and when he loses this on retirement he's apt to feel emasculated. It is esp-ecially difficult for newly retired working-class men who still have younger wives going out to work and supplementing the meagre family income. Many older working-class men feel a sense of humiliation when they find that they're expected to do housework and numerous tasks that they have regarded as "women's work". In what way can they now assert their masculinity? In masculine sports? But they've lost their former physical vigour. In bed? But their potency has declined and they may blame sexual failures on the decreased attractiveness of their wives.

Although nowadays there's probably little difference between the sexual practices of the working-class and middle-class as far as young people are concerned, the sort of sexual techniques that are described in modern sex-manuals were almost unknown to working class people 40 years ago when these older couples formed their sexual unions, and indeed many men would have been quite shocked if their wives had behaved in bed "like whores". Middle-class couples are less constrained by the conventions of sex-role division and hence they don't suffer on retirement from the same degree of stress. Also, although attitudes to sexual practices are conditioned by numerous complex factors of upbringing, the "sexual revolution" affected the middle-class earlier.

Are Men harder hit than Women?

Men may be specially vulnerable in one respect: they retire five years later than women, which is utterly ridiculous as older women are generally tougher and live longer. The man may expect to see a great deal more of his wife when he retires, whether she's had a job or worked in the home. However, long before he's retired, many women whose children have left home have filled their days with various activities outside the house, and developed circles of friends who have nothing to do with their husband's world. He therefore feels rejected and left out in the marital home; his status as a worker is not replaced by any sort of status as was implied by the outworn concept of "the head of the household". If he's retired expecting to have a pleasant time pottering around the house being looked after by his loving wife, he may be shocked to find what appears to be a rather different woman living in the house: one who's very busy with her own concerns, who has a host of day-time friends, and has really no more time to give to him than was customary when he was working. She may be as good in bed as ever, but when resentments spring up between couples, the giving and witholding of sex may be used as a weapon to punish and establish mastery. The power-struggle again.

It hardly needs saying that the retirement of the man may present special problems for the wife. A man who is out at work for most of the day, with his energies largely absorbed by such work, may be a quite tolerable partner to live with, but when he's around all the time she may find him a real pain. She may feel that now she's living with a different man. "How did I ever put up with him before?" she wonders. Again, the marital bed may become the battleground in an emotional and sexual sense over issues that were not primarily sexual at all. Years of very minor sexual frustration on both sides may now become the subject of bitter recrimination. The power-struggle again! Add to all this the greatly reduced family income on retirement which is the lot of so many working-class people, and we have a nice can of worms.

What am I arguing – that couples ought to split up when they reach retirement? No, but the problems should be fully understood and even anticipated. We come back to Alex Comfort's statement, "We can only alter the manipulative cost-accountancy concept of retirement ... by changing society". So how do we change society?

The Future of Retirement

As noted above, people are retiring earlier, and early retirement may become a matter of social policy, encouraging or even forcing people to give up work at below the statutory age. In the U.S.A. the United Auto Workers offer inducement for people to retire at the age of fifty-five, if they undertake to leave the industry. It has been estimated that by the year 2050 most manual workers will have a working life of only twenty years, and such a prospect is seriously offered as a palliative for unemployment. Of course one can't take such projections into the future entirely seriously, as conditions are changing so rapidly in the modern world. It is of interest, however, to study the way people in positions of power and influence are thinking. I do not, myself, subscribe to the conspiracy theory of politics, or believe that the "ruling class" are a lot of bastards intent on enriching themselves by grinding the faces of the poor, but I do think that perfectly idiotic social policies can be forced on us if we don't see the issues clearly and fight to ensure a better society for the future.

In an earlier chapter I remarked that a neurosurgeon can't work with the required degree of skill much after the age of fifty, or a coal-heaver (are there such people nowadays?) heave coal as effectively after that age. But no-one is just a neurosurgeon or a coal-heaver. Our present job does not define us as a person, and we don't become an un-person when we retire from it.

Age Discrimination at Work.

The governmental view on the employment of older people is highly inconsistent, and we may note a changing tune as the General Elections of the 1990s approach, as the older section of the population have considerable voting power. In 1984, Peter Morrison, who was then a Minister of State for Employment, stated that:

> the government is not convinced that legislating against age discrimination in employment would be beneficial or practicable. We recognize the value of the experience, skill and other qualities that older workers bring to their jobs and we hope that employers will keep their employment practices under review[2]

Try reading the above passage substituting "sex discrimination" or "racial discrimination", and consider how it sounds!

We don't see nowadays advertisements of vacant positions which add "No blacks need apply", but it's taken for granted that employers should be free to set their own ageist standards. The Equal Opportunities Commission monitored 11,373 job advertisements across a range of periodicals, Over 25 per cent of these advertisements stated an age preference. Almost all specified the age of *45 or under*, and 65 per cent of those mentioning age gave a limit of 35 or under[3]. Similarly, a study of jobs advertised in papers such as the *Sunday Times, Daily Telegraph, Financial Times* and *Guardian*, showed that 88.5 per cent mentioned an age limit of 40[4]. So you thought that you'd only encounter ageist discrimination when you reached your sixties did you?

If an employer wishes to see pretty young girls around the works, rather than women with wrinkles, he's entitled to sack all the women over what is "the normal retiring age" for the job. This is lawful, and he's not in breach of contract. This normal retiring age varies with the work, and is generally around 60, but a woman over that age who is perfectly efficient at her job, and who needs the money, can simply be sacked if that is the employer's whim. Peter Morrison's hope that "employers will keep their their employment practices under review" can be answered by some employers with the private resolve, "Yes, and we'll find means if we can, of getting rid of all those old bags over 40 too!"

By 1988 the government were still defending their ageist policies regarding employment and recruitment, and a Department of Employment memorandum reads.

> There is currently no legislation in this country to prevent age discrimination in employment and the Government's view is that it would be neither beneficial nor practical to do so. Employers should be free to recruit the most suitable workers and not be restricted from doing so by legislation or regulation[5].

The above statement implies that employers always know who are the most suitable workers, but it is notorious that they don't. What does "suitable" mean – suitable to please the boss or suitable to get the work done? The negative stereotypes of older people that have been explored at some length in this book affect employers as much as anyone else. In addition, there's the cruel fact that a great deal of work needs only minimal skill of a huge number of employees, so it doesn't really matter what sex, colour or age they are. A prejudiced employer might like to get rid of all the blacks from his works, saying, "Darkies are lazy – everybody knows that!", but as things are, he can only exercise his prejudices in the matter of age.

Not all firms have employment policies that are governed by whim and prejudice. Some firms such as Tesco have adopted a policy of keeping on older people and recruiting others because their own experience shows that they have a better work-record than younger workers, and a smaller labour turnover. British Rail would formerly only take younger workers up to their middle twenties for training as drivers – a practice for which there was no reason other than a false assumption about age, trainability and skill. Now they take workers up to their middle forties for training as drivers.

As mentioned above, the approaching General Elections of the 1990s have caused a significant change in the tune of governmental statements. Norman Fowler has said:

> We are challenging the whole concept that retirement ages should get earlier and earlier. It should be left to individuals to decide when to retire .... The present 60/65 fixed retirement ages are totally misconceived .... There is going to be much greater scope for people to continue their careers for much longer, and greater value will be placed on their experience than ever before[6].

He did not add, "So vote Tory all you wrinklies!", but this was his message.

From time to time the number of millions unemployed is announced by Tweedle-Dee in office, and challenged by a few hundred thousand by Tweedle-Dum out of office, but both sides know how grossly the figures mis-represent the true picture. They get rid of a huge section of unemployed from the figures announced by calling them "Retired", and they know that this is increasing year by year.

Towards a Sane Policy on Work.

Throughout our lives, our capacities change. Put very crudely, we get less physically robust with ageing but we get far more experienced. It is absurd to imagine that an individual will make his or her best contribution to society by staying in the same job for a lifetime. This is recognized to a great extent in the academic world and in the professions, but it is a matter of social injustice that in all forms of work there should not be a similar recognition. We are moving out of the past era when it was considered natural that the "labouring class" should be worked to exhaustion as long as they could stand the pace, and then put out to grass for a few years before they died. What I am proposing is nothing very new; writers such as William Morris in his *Useful Work Versus Useless Toil*, and Kropotkin in his *The Wage System* were proposing much the same thing over a century ago. Now we have come through an extraordinary period in which a secular religion, Marxist-Leninism, has dominated revolutionary social theorizing. It is true that Fabianism has been its great rival, and much favoured by establishment intellectuals, and I remember that F.A. Ridley summarized Nazism very pithily – "Simply Fabianism in jack boots". But the shocking disaster of this secular religion in practice that we have witnessed may initiate a new era of re-thinking.

What should we seek to do about the institution of retirement? We should seek to abolish it. So are we to work all our lives? Yes, why not? Providing the activity known as "work" is useful, interesting and creative, and suited to our individual capacities, it will grace our lives whether we be eighteen or eighty, but for this to be so we must envisage some fundamental changes in the economic basis of our society. Let us be quite clear about the nature of the great bulk of work that is performed in our society today. Most work is pretty terrible whether it can be classed as white-collar or blue-collar, and most people go to work reluctantly simply because they need the wages. Terkel's book *Working*[7] reports on what a great variety of people say about their jobs:

> For the many, there's hardly concealed discontent. The blue-collar blues is not more bitterly sung than the white-collar moan. "I'm a machine," says the spot-welder. "I'm caged," says the bank teller, and echoes the hotel clerk. "I'm a mule," says the steel worker. "A monkey can do what I do," says the receptionist. "I'm less than a farm impliment" says the migrant worker. "I'm an object," says the high-fashion model. Blue-collar and white-collar call upon the identical phrase, "I'm a robot."

It is obvious therefore, that the great bulk of workers today will totally reject the concept of the abolition of retirement, at least, when they are in the midst of the daily grind. But when unemployed on the dole, or unemployed for life (retired) they may think twice about it, for as well as the wages, employment gives them the company of their work-mates, some sense of purpose, and some hope of advancement. This is so huge a subject that I can't do better than to refer the reader to the excellent Freedom Press publication *Why Work?*, a collection of 32 essays by various writers[8].

Chapter 7: Notes

1. Alex Comfort, *A Good Age*. Pan Books, 1989.
2. Questions in Parliament. *Employment Gazette*, 1984, 92, 31, H.M.S.O.
3. F. Laczko & C. Phillipson, "Defending the right ot work". *Age: The Unrecognized Discrimination*. Age Concern, 1990.
4. P. Naylor, "In praise of older workers", *Personenel Management,* 1987, November, 44-48.
5. House of Commons Employment Committee (Session 1988-89 *The Employment Patterns of the Over 50s*, Vol. 11. H.M.S.O.
6. *Sunday Times* 29th January, 1989.
7. S. Terkel, *Working: People Talk About What They Do And How they Feel About What They Do*. Pantheon, 1974.
8. *Why Work*. Freedom Press, 1983.

Looking to the Future:
A Libertarian Perspective

As was mentioned in Chapter 6, a totally new factor has entered human society, the emergence of a numerically substantial group of people in the later decades of life who are relatively fit and active, and less and less prepared to accept the low status and relative powerlessness that has been traditionally assigned to "the old". These people are in a period of life that has come to be known as the Third Age by a number of recent writers such as Peter Laslett[1].

The outstanding anomaly is that people in the Third Age, who may well have an active life of about thirty years, are supposed to be "retired", and are treated as such both in law and in custom. Not only is this the present reality of the population structure, but the position is certainly going to be more and more exaggerated as time goes on. Table 8.1 shows the position as it is now and how it will be in 40 years time.

TABLE 8.1

GREAT BRITAIN

Comparison between the "dependent" and the "working" population. Figures in thousands. Percentages of total population shown.

	1991	%	2031	%
Children below 16 years	11336	20.2	11854	19.9
Adults now retired	10291	18.4	14166	23.8
(males 65+; females 60+)				
Total dependents	21627	38.6	26020	43.7
Working population	34360	61.4	33592	56.3
(Age 16 to retirement)				

Source: Office of Population Censuses and Surveys (1987) *Population Projections by the Government Actuary PP2. No 16.* London: H.M.S.O.

First it should be noted that in 1991 there was a substantial proportion (18.4%) of the population officially "retired", and therefore theoretically dependent on the "working" population (of whom a great number are unemployed at present). At this date the number of children, (who are also "dependents"), was greater than the "retired", but in 40 years time the position will be reversed; so as time goes on and these children become the "working" population, the latter will have shrunk proportionally. In 1991 the ratio of "working" to "retired" was 3.33/1; in the year 2031 the proportion will be 2.37/1, and the trend will inevitably continue in this direction..

The above figures are subject to all sorts of ifs and buts, and we don't really know what is going to happen to the world in future history. However, they should alert us to the fact that what has already happened to society in the twentieth century is going to be made progressively more extreme as time goes on. The Third Age has come to stay. Medical science now enables older people not only to live longer, but to continue to be fit and active practically until the day they drop dead, so the whole concept of retirement becomes progressively more ridiculous. The "new old", as they have been called, are not going to behave like older people in former times; they have already begun to demand more power in society, a better standard of living, and to continue to enjoy full adult status. No longer do they hoard what capital they have, large or small, in order that their inheritors will benefit; they are spending it, or at least conserving it less strictly than in earlier times. The result will be that in the future wealth will progressively become social rather than personal.

All the above is now becoming apparent to social scientists, but looking back in our immediate history, social and political theorists of both the left and the right, were entirely unaware of the great changes that were taking place in society. Their theories are now outmoded because they did not take note of such inevitable and significant changes that were already in operation. The introduction of the widespread use of contraception affecting one end of the age-scale, and the vast improvement in public health affecting the other end of the age-scale, have had a profound effect on the population structure of the developed nations of the world, and the Third World nations will inevitably follow. We are told that the world is witnessing a population explosion, but this is partly due to older people living longer, and not just to the reduction of infant mortality. Sooner or later births are going to be limited in the Third World, despite the preaching of such reactionary figures as Pope John Paul. As there becomes a larger and larger proportion of the population in the later decades of life, so the proportion of the population in the procreative years becomes smaller and smaller; thus the problem in some countries may be that there are not enough children growing up to be recruited into the working population. Or will it be, as I have suggested, that the whole adult population will be working whatever their age, in the sense that they will be actively productive of goods and services?

The Effect on Man-Woman Relationships

Another great change has come about in society due to the emergence of the Third Age. The excess of women over men in the later decades of life has become more and more pronounced. This is because women tend to live about seven years longer than men. Why this is so is still a matter of conjecture. It may be a natural feature of our species, for the same phenomenon occurs in some other animal species. Table 8.2 shows the population figures for the year 1987.

TABLE 8.2.

Estimated Population in England and Wales for the Year 1987

Thousands

Age	Total Males	Females	Married Males	Females	Unmarried* Males	Females	Female Excess:
50-54	1334.8	1333.4	1105.0	1071.5	229.8	261.9	42.1
55-59	1319.1	1360.6	1090.6	1035.8	228.5	324.8	96.3
60-64	1270.6	1376.3	1041.3	942.0	229.3	434.3	205.0
65-69	1120.6	1328.0	905.3	775.7	215.3	552.3	337.0
70-74	869.0	1170.9	666.0	522.5	203.0	648.4	445.0
75+	1143.2	2240.7	82.6	496.2	1060.6	1744.5	683.9

* The status of the "Unmarried" is single + widowed + divorced
: The figure for "Excess" is derived by subtracting the figure for unmarried males from that of unmarried females.

Statistics derived from Table 1.1. *Office of Population Studies: Series FM2 No.14*, H.M.S.O.

It will be observed from the last column of Table 8.2 that the excess of *single* women over *single* men increases steadily after the age of 50 so that there are as many as 1,809,300 women (the total of the column) who could not be paired with a single male partner in their own age group, either in marriage or in any monogamous relationship. Some writers[2] have suggested that in the later years of life people should form polygamous relationships, one man having several wives or mistresses simultaneously. There is one important objection to such an idea: while a man in youth or middle-age may service several women sexually, this is not feasible later on as it is normal for men to lose their sexual drive and capacity at a greater rate than women as the ageing process proceeds. Since a great number of women are rendered single in later life by bereavement and divorce, and some are not happy with this celibate state, we might have expected that the feminist movement would have been actively concerned about it. Some feminists would dispense with marriage and male-female co-habitation altogether, and some, such as Kearon[3] are self-confessed man-haters, and make their hatred quite explicit. Unfortunately these younger radical feminists appear to be concerned only with the problems of those in their own generation. So far they have made little effort to address themselves to the problems of women in later life. They should be concerned that one day they themselves will be elderly and living in a society that is significantly different from that which they experience today. Barbara Macdonald[4], a feminist campaigner who is now in her 70s, describes how she has come to be rejected by the younger members of the women's movement because they assume that at her age she can no longer be regarded as a relevant and valuable "sister".

Another elderly feminist writer puts the case for older single women simply ceasing to consider the relevance of men in their lives. She writes:

> Over three million of us are widows. I feel that most of us have spent most of our lives in a close relationship and would prefer to live this way. Sometimes a feeling of loyalty to our lost partners or lack of confidence in ourselves leads to a withdrawal from society, and I am all in favour of any measure which helps to bring us back to life.
>
> However, even given the confidence and desire to venture forth and meet new people, there are serious obstacles ahead. First is the shortage of men, a discrepancy between the sexes that increases with age..... Nothing is sadder than the pages of advertisements in, for example, SAGA Magazine, where the number

of women so heavily outnumbers the number of men seeking new partners or even social contacts. We are all familiar with social occasions where men are a rarity, overwhelmed by crowds of women. The same applies to holiday trips. And it is not going to get any better.

Of course there are some men around, even after eliminating those who are already married or seriously unfit. But there are still problems ahead. Gold diggers and con men have a field day, but can usually be spotted in time. More tricky is the "hot meals and slippers syndrome"; those men who are really looking for an unpaid nurse/housekeeper for "their old age". Fortunately for them, there are many women who relish such a role, but at least both sides should realize where they stand.

I am all in favour of a realistic approach. Of course one can fall in love at any age and have that love reciprocated. Such people are extremely fortunate and I wish them all the best. But surely it is a waste of precious days left to us not to realize the odds against finding another partner and to face up to life alone....

We are the first generation to exist in such large numbers in our age group. The life style of our elders no longer applies, but we are the ones who have to forge new paths. No one can do it for us. For women alone the adaptation is hard but surely not impossible. If love or friendship comes your way, that's a bonus, but meanwhile it's no use repining. We need to summon all the resources we can to build a new and creative life. Only when we value ourselves will society value us too.[4]

The Lesbian Alternative

One alternative that the above writer doesn't consider is the formation of lesbian sexual relationships in later life between women who have previously been exclusively heterosexual. There's now quite a body of contemporary literature discussing lesbianism, much of it being written by feminists who regard it as a natural alternative for those who don't wish to be involved sexually with men. As there's a great shortage of available men in the later decades of life, it would seem that there's a reasonable case for single women forming lesbian associations with one another.

When many men are deprived of female company it's well known that they turn rather easily to homosexual behaviour, as in prisons, the navy, and other all-male communities. Although much the same thing happens in convents, boarding schools etc., the tendency is far less pronounced for women. The Kinsey studies, and all subsequent surveys of human sexuality, have shown a far greater prevalence of homosexual behaviour among men than among women. In the extensive survey of Brecher[5] of the sexual behaviour of men and women over 50, 301 (13%) of the men admitted to having had homosexual relationships, but only 131 (8%) of the women admitted this. This survey also asked the question "Have you ever felt sexually attracted to a person of your own gender?" Here, rather surprisingly, more women than men admitted to having felt *homosexual attraction*. Brecher seeks to explain these findings in terms of the very different upbringings that girls and boys experienced in the earlier part of this century when they were young, the girls having been subjected to stronger taboos about sex. It may be that in the next century, older women, having experienced more liberal treatment in childhood, and having lived in a society that is fairly tolerant of homosexual behaviour, will be more prone to form lesbian relationships if they are rendered single.

Developments need not stop there. Above, it was pointed out that the usual sort of polygamous relationship would be impractical for people in later life because older women have greater sexual drive and capacity than men of comparable age. But some women might well take to a bi-sexual way of life, having both male and female lovers, for as has been stressed throughout the present book, the concept of sexuality needs to be broadened considerably from that which we have inherited from our Victorian ancestors.

The Revolt of the Old

The title above is that which heads the last chapter of the Starr-Weiner Report which has been mentioned earlier in the present book. Anyone can indulge in arm-chair speculation for the future, but we should pay more attention to those who have done considerable research with older people. The authors of this Report pedict the following changes:

> The later years possess many potential hazards: loss of friends and relations, loneliness, disenfranchisement, economic vulnerability, to name just a few. All these reflect on one's personal worth and power. Sex and power, as we have noted, are intertwined so that sexuality will be influenced by the overall status of older people....

Unlike the present generation of the elderly who are largely copers and adapters, future generations are likely to be doers and shapers. Rather than moulding their own behavior and needs to conform to a given reality, they will be more likely to alter the environment to fit their needs. Freed of the stereotypes of what an old person should be, dedicated to personal fulfilment and convinced of the power of people to unite in shaping their world, they will *act* not react. They will come up with solutions and alternatives that will change the face of the later years.[6]

Has a New "Class" Emerged?

We may consider whether a new "class" has emerged in society, and, harking back to Wilhelm Reich, whether the social tensions are to be viewed in terms of "class struggle". Here we are using a Marxist concept, and it is likely that Marx himself would not have agreed that the people in the Third Age constitute a "class", for he was concerned with socio-economic classes represented by the "proletariat" and the "bourgeoisie", but people in the Third Age include both the "haves" and the "have-nots". However, writers later than Marx, such as E.P. Thompson, have advanced a more sophisticated view of "class":

> class happens when some men, as a result of common experiences (inherited or shared), feel and articulate the identity of their interests as between themselves and as against other men whose interests are different from (and usually opposed to) theirs[8]

Obviously, within any sort of "class" there will be important individual differences, and these differences will militate against solidarity and class-consciousness. Thus in Marx's "proletariat" there were differences based on age, sex, trade, ethnic origin etc., which were divisive, just as among people in the present-day Third Age the possession or non-possession of property is an important factor that cuts across feelings of identity of interest. Indeed, if individuals are sufficiently rich, the usual attributes of the old hardly apply. They retain a great deal of their power, and, interestingly enough, as power and sexuality are strongly connected, they can defy society's strictures against the sexuality of the old with impunity, particularly if they are male. There are plenty of examples of rich old men acquiring young wives or mistresses, and it being entirely socially acceptable. However, if a retired manual worker took a young mistress to live with him it is unlikely that they would be accepted by the local working-class community; it is likely that they would condemn him as a "dirty old man". For an elderly working-class woman to take on a young toy-boy would also invite ostracism.

Reich, and more conventional Marxist writers, have had a great deal to say about ideology. Ira Cohen, a commentator on Reich, writes:

> To counteract the effects of ideology, the exploited class should be encouraged to understand the conditions of the existing social structure in terms of their own interests. This could lead them to recognize the possibility that they could transform the class structure through their own actions. It is this understanding that Lukacs referred to with the phrase "imputed class consciousness." The development of class relationships within capitalism makes the emergence of this consciousness possible[9].

What has been described in the present book as the prevailing "myth" about "the old" is, of course a ruling ideology, just as there are racist and sexist ideologies. The writers who are striving to break down the myth and to emancipate older people from its dominance, such as Alex Comfort[10], Starr and Weiner[11,] Edward Brecher[12], and Butler and Lewis[13], are trying to replace the dominant ideology with a new one, and create a new consciousness for the emergent "class" of people in the Third Age.

In her commentary on Reich, Ira Cohen continues:

> The idea of people assuming responsibility for their own lives marks Reich's contribution to the concept of class consciousness. It must be emphasised that this is a responsibility which is to be exercised in every sphere of life. The authority of civil society or the state is no more legitimate than the authority of property. Humans must consciously organize their lives in accordance with their desires and instincts. Tradition finds virtue in discipline and self-denial; against these, Reich argued, the revolution "must set the principle of happiness and abundance on earth." Reich was fully convinced that a free society could be based only on the satisfaction of human's instinctual needs..... Economic problems are not the only ones which trouble people, nor is economic dependency the only or even most significant conservative force in people's lives. Repression of erotic desires, family ties, the very structure of the family and identification with other symbols of authority all serve as buttresses of the status quo[14].

Here Cohen is commenting on how far Reich differed from orthodox Marxism, and indeed, as many people have commented, at
one period of his varied career he came very close to an anarchist
view of society.

Economic Privation in Later Life

Although the "class" of people in the Third Age contains both rich
and poor, and this constitutes an obstacle to the development of
an appropriate class-consciousness, we should not be unaware that
for a huge number of people the nact of ageing means poverty. The
better-off minority are humourously referred to as the "Woopies"
(Well Off Older People) and the "Jollies (Jet-setting Oldies with
Lots of Loot), but the conspicuous nature of the free-spending
section of the older population should not blind us to the more
general standard of living for retired people at present.

The plain fact is that most people over pensionable age are living
in considerably straightened circumstances. In the Welfare State,
poverty is still with us, and most poor people are poor because they
are elderly. Taking the figures of the Department of Social Security
which are for very recent years, about a million pensioners have
been living on incomes below the poverty line of the
Supplementary Benefit. We may ask why, in a formal dem-
ocracy such as we have in Britain, so many older people put up
with living out the rest of their lives in poverty? Their penury is
reflected in all sorts of measures of deprivation as shown in various
surveys.[15] They are inadequately housed; they lack proper heating
in cold weather; their diet is poor, and they show a lack of consumer
durables. Various forms of disability are more common in later
life among poorer people, and we've already seen how the numbers
in the most vulnerable elderly group will greatly increase in the
coming century. Being somewhat disabled costs money. Evidence
published by the Office of Population Censuses and Surveys[16]
indicated that pensioners with minor disabilities needed to pay
an extra £5.70 per week, and those with severe disabilities spent
an extra £10.50 a week. This was in 1985, but some have claimed
that these figures greatly underestimate the true extent to which
disability among pensioners involves extra expenditure[17].

Britain is not a particularly poor country among others of the
European community, yet pensioners here are considerably worse
off. Among nine member countries of the EEC Britain came second
to last in the standard of living of pensioners[18]. The purchasing
power of a single person's pension in Britain is only 50% of that of

the Dutch pensioner, 60% of the West German pensioner, and less than 75% of the French. Whatever may be the cause of these differences between the European countries, the attitude of the British towards their own poverty is reflected in the fact that, according to the Department of Social Security, in 1985 900,000 people failed to claim the benefits to which they were entitled, and this applied particularly to Supplementary Benefit - 79% of elderly people who were entitled to it failed to claim it[19]. Is this due to irrational pride, to apathetic acceptance of poverty, or mainly to a strong revulsion from having any truck with bureaucracy? The spectre of Mr Bumble the beadle still haunts the poorer people of this country. People have grown up to expect to be poorer in later life and to have to stint themselves a bit as they get older, but there's no reason why this should be. Why shouldn't everybody expect a *greater* degree of affluence in later life?

The spectre of the Poor Law, tempered by beneficent private charity, still haunts the people who were born in the early decades of this century. It's patronizing to allow older persons various "concessions". For instance, they are allowed to travel at a lower rate on public transport - provided they travel at the correct time of day - but wouldn't it be more in keeping with their dignity and conception of their value as citizens, if they had a decent income and hence could afford to pay the same as all other adults? The spirit of the much-parodied Victorian poem *'Twas Christmas Day in the Workhouse* still finds expression in the £10 tip that is given to pensioners at Christmas time.

Commenting on the poverty and supineness of elderly people in Britain, Mike Bender writes:

There are a variety of reasons:

There is no reason why they should be politically united, as the elderly are as variegated as the younger members of society. To deny this is to resort to stereotyping — they're all the same. However, one might have thought that they could unite in wanting decent pensions.

There is a heavy over-representation of women who are generally less assertive than men, especially for the age cohort (born 1900-1930).[20]

But Bender does not attempt to tackle the question of why pensioners in Britain are so much more supine than those in other European countries. This is indeed a difficult and complex question, but it may partly relate to the fact that those in the Third Age in Britain are still suffering from the hang-over of the Victorian era. Queen Victoria's reign saw Britain as the dominant imperial power in the world, the country that led the world in sexual repression, in prudery and hypocrisy, often to the amazement of foreigners. According to Freud, and to his follower Reich, sexual repression is the price we pay for a society that is organized for political and military dominance. I do not say that this is the whole answer, or that the model is at all complete, but I am reminded that Sparta was eventually dominant over the comparatively liberal and much more civilized state of Athens.

Regarding the relative supineness of the elderly in Britain, it should be noted that all the pioneers mentioned earlier who are striving to create a new ideology for the Third Age are American, with the exception of Alex Comfort; but he was working in America during the period of his life when he wrote *A Good Age*. Britain has, at present, no equivalent of the Grey Panthers, the body that is striving for the rights of older people in America. Are we about to see, here and abroad, an effective "Revolt of the Old", as suggested above by Starr and Weiner? This present book can do little more than to try to present a libertarian view of our rapidly changing society, and the position of older people in it, to combat the traditional stereotype of the elderly, and to indicate directions in which society may change.

What about "Love"?

The word "love" is at the beginning of the title of my book, and I use it advisedly. Chapter 5 discusses progress towards a new concept of sexuality, a concept that certainly embraces love, and in no sentimental sense. It does not matter whether a relationship is of very long standing, or is a brief "shipboard romance", or just a one-night stand, what is being celebrated in the best sense of sexuality is *love of life*, expressed in the consummation of the attraction between two people. I cannot do better than to quote the great Jewish writer Bashevis Singer:

> The love of the old and the middle-aged is a theme that is recurring more and more in my works of fiction. Literature has neglected the old and their emotions. The novelists never told us that in love, as in other matters, the young are just beginners, and that the art of love matures with age and experience. Furthermore, while many of the young believe that the world can be made better

by sudden changes in the social order and by bloody and exhausting revolutions, most older people have learnt that hatred and cruelty never produce anything but their own kind. The only hope of mankind is love in its various forms and manifestations - the source of them all being love of life, which, as we know, increases and ripens with the years.[21]

Some people may think that the above passage smacks of sentimentality, but all who are familiar with the works of Singer will know that he is the least sentimental of writers, and is utterly realistic in his portrayal of life. Much of the libertarian literature of the past has celebrated the military achievements of such revolutionary figures as Zapata, Mahkno, and Durruti, but these heroic figures inspired their followers, and those who have admired them elsewhere, not on grounds of sheer military efficiency but because of the broad humanity that inspired the movements that they led. With hindsight, we know where the "bloody and exhausting revolutions" of the past have led, but where dreadful tyrannies have eventually been overthrown, it is to the love of life of ordinary people that the credit must be given.

I have grown old along with my generation and have witnessed changes in the direction of greater liberality, tolerance and understanding against the rather ugly background of the times into which I was born. It is my hope that Bashevis Singer is right that loving, in its broadest sense, love of life, rather than attachment to power over others, wealth or religion, matures with age and the older societies of the future will accordingly achieve the better society for which revolutionary libertarians have striven towards for so long.

Chapter 8: Notes

1. Peter Laslett, op. cit. Chap. 6.

2. See V. Kassel, "Polygyny after 60." In K.C.W. Kammeyer (ed.) *Confronting the Issues*. Allyn & Bacon, 1975.

3. P. Kearon, "man-hating." In *Notes from the Second Year*, cited by J. Bernard, *The Future of Marriage*. Yale University Press, 1970,

4. B. Macdonald & C. Rich, *Look me in the Eye: Old Women, Ageing and Ageism*. The Women's Press, 1985.

5. J.T. Personal communication to the author.

6. E.M. Brecher, Love, Sex and Aging: A Concumer Union Report. Little, Brown & Co., 1984.

7. B.D. Starr & M.B. Weiner, *The Starr-Weiner Report on Sex and Sexuality in the Mature Years*. McGraw Hill, 1981.

8. E.P. Thompson, *The Making of the English Working Class*. Penguin Books, 1968.

9. I. Cohen, *Reich, Freud and Marx*. New York University Press, 1982.

10. Alex Comfort, op. cit. Introduction.

11. B.D. Starr & M.B. Weiner, op. cit. Introduction.

12. E. Brecher, op. cit. Introduction.

13. R.N. Butler & M.I. Lewis, op. cit. Introduction.

14. I. Cohen, op. cit. above.

15. See J. Mack & S. Lansley, *Poor Britain*. Allen & Unwin, 1985.

16. See J. Martin, H. Meltzer & D. Elliott, *The Prevalence of Disability Among Adults. Report I.* H.M.S.O. 1988.

17. See P. Thompson, J. Buckle & M. Lavery, *Not in the OPCS Survey*. Disability Income Group, 1988.

18. See K. Chapman, "Looking around Europe". *Eurolink Age Bullitin*, March 1990.

19. Department of Social Security, *Supplementary Benefit Take-up 1985/86: Technical Note* 1989.

20. M. Bender, "Elderly depression: acting out society's unresolved conflicts." *PSIGE Neswsletter*, 1991-92, No. 41.

21. I. Bashevis Singer, op. cit. above.

APPENDIX: Further Reading

R.N. Butler & M.I. Lewis, *Love and Sex After 60*. Revised Edition. Harper & Row, 1989. £5.50.

An excellent guide to all spects of sexuality in later life, with discussion of the personal and social implications.

I. Cohen, *Marx, Freud and Reich*. New York University Press, 1982.

This book puts a lot of Reich's early and more important ideas rather more lucidly than Reich put them himself, and traces his relationship with the Marxist movement of his time.

Alex Comfort, *A Good Age*. Pan Books, 1990.

This book just about covers everything concerning sexuality and power in modern society as they affect older people. Alex Comfort is now a most respected figure of international repute in the study of ageing, as well as having made a significant contribution to sexology. His writing has lost nothing of the vigour and wit that characterized his earlier anarchist writings. £5.95.

H.B. Gibson, *The Emotional and Sexual Lives of Older People*. Chapman & Hall, 1991, £13.95.

This book is really directed to health-care professionals, such as nurses, doctors, clinical psychologists, social workers etc., and hence may be a bit heavy going in places for the average reader, but it contains a great wealth of information.

W. Greengross & S. Greengross, *Living, Loving and Ageing*. Age Concern, 1989. £4.95.

This is written for "the average reader" and contains a lot of common-sense advice about sexuality in later life.. It is fairly elementary and does not deal with contentious social issues.

E. McEwen, (ed.), *Age: The Unrecognised Discrimination*. Age Concern, 1990. £9.95

This is a collection of 8 essays by various writers on various aspects of ageist discrimination in contemporary society. It is well worth your while to ask your local library to get it

W. Reich, *The Mass Psychology of Fascism*.

This is an English translation of the original book. It is very dated, but it sets out the original thesis. See I. Cohen above.

W. Reich, Sexpol: Essays 1929-34. £12.00.

This is obtainable from Freedom Press.

WHY WORK ?
ARGUMENTS FOR THE LEISURE SOCIETY

Third printing 1990

The title of this collection by various writers, past and present, is meant to be provocative. What this volume does not attempt to do is to solve the problems of capitalism which can only be solved by abolishing the system of production for profit and putting in its place production for needs. Here the distinction is made between work and employment, between useful work and useless toil, between pleasurable work and boring, well-paid, useless employment.

The contributors to this volume range from William Morris with his ever topical essay on *Useful Work versus Useless Toil* which was first published more than a hundred years ago, new translations of Kropotkin's *Wage System* and Camillo Berneri's *The Problem of Work*, to contemporary writers who all draw the same conclusions as Lewis Mumford in *Technics and Civilization* (now available as a Freedom Press title) when he declared more than fifty years ago:

"No working ideal for machine production can be based solely on the gospel of work; still less can it be based upon an uncritical belief in constantly raising the quantitative standard of consumption. If we are to achive a purposive and cultivated use of the enormous energies now happily at out disposal, we must examine in detail the processes that lead up to the final state of leisure., free activity, creation."

Tony Gibson contributes a mini-classic to this volume with the title "Who will do the Dirty Work?"

£4.50   210 pages   ISBN 0 900384 25 5

The Employment Question and other Essays

by
Denis Pym

The author writes:

"In these essays I question the legitimacy of employing institutions and, in particular, the monopoly we give them in the creation of wealth. This does not mean I am against employing institutions but I am against our dependence on the corporate world which is typical of our relations with a wide range of artifacts from the printed word, to television and the motor-car. As I see it, we need to take back into ourselves the authority for decision and action. In western industrial societies, people most clearly act on behalf of themselves in that domain we typically dismiss as 'The Black Economy'. This emerging community economy is part of a dual system. The aspect we currently write large as the formal economy is for machines and will employ decreasing numbers of people. The other, founded on home and community, offers people the opportunity to reunite their social and economic lives and use the tools and techniques which suit their personal and social requirements."

68 pages   ISBN 0 900384 31 X   £2